Great Necessities

A Gaucher Memoir

Wayne D. Rosenfield, Ph.D.

8/15/2015

To Brian Trial —
Be well. Stay strong!

Wayne Rosenfield

To Sue, Aaron, David, George, and Muriel Rosenfield, who have been at my side through these events. My story is also your story.

Preface

I have had many opportunities to speak publicly about my personal experiences with Gaucher Disease. I have presented my story at professional meetings, in classes for students of medicine and engineering, and at meetings of national advocacy organizations. I have spoken at the invitation of pharmaceutical companies to some of their employees. A consortium of pharmaceutical companies once asked me to provide a briefing for certain members of the US Congress. I have spoken publicly in four different countries about my experiences, and for one meeting in the United States that was streamed live over the Internet to a global audience. I'm not a natural-born orator, and I worked hard to develop a presentation style that can be enjoyable and informative for the listeners.

As with any speech, the most credible presentation would come from someone who knows his subject matter. I don't need to study a script prior to lecturing about this story. I simply describe my experiences. I lived this story, and I still do. The manner in which I speak about my experiences is flavored by my sometimes-wry view of everyday life and by my great personal enjoyment of humor. Some of these personal characteristics became, perhaps accidentally, assets in my survival of some very great challenges.

The relaxed, humorous presentation style that I have tried to develop, with some success, may understate the intensity of the difficulty faced by someone in a very big struggle. It's hard at such times to see that a good outcome is possible. But the result, I think, is that I can present myself as a role model for coping, victory, and hope for people who are now in their own great struggles.

I have met many people in my professional life, separate from my Gaucher Disease narrative, who do not see coping and victory as realistically attainable for themselves. I have known many people who lost their hope for a future that is better than the present. I think I know what they feel. I have serendipitously, through life experience, found a path that worked for me.

This book is not a manual for self directed therapy. This is a narrative of the lessons from my own experience, and how I improvised my survival. It was only in retrospect that I fully realized how my thinking and behavior during my worst times resembled elements of cognitive behavioral therapy.

In recent years I have met dozens of individuals and families affected by Gaucher Disease. Sometimes I run into old friends at a treatment center, and sometimes I meet people who, like me, are attending a larger meeting. Occasionally a pharmaceutical company asks me to present a condensed version of my Gaucher Disease experience. This gives me the opportunity to meet people affected by Gaucher Disease in pleasant venues. We're able to chat and share each other's company over lunch or dinner. I have learned through experience that many people hearing my story have found it to be useful for themselves in their own journeys. Some people have asked me for more detail. The problem is that in short encounters I don't have the opportunity to fully relate the details of my story and its lessons. Perhaps the support that I try to provide personally can be conveyed through a book, with a completeness that is not possible through other means.

The story contains my exposure to some of the most exemplary and, at times, substandard examples of professional behavior. But it is a story primarily about me. The specific individuals named in this story have given me their consent to be identified personally in my narrative. I refer to other individuals only with fictitious names and descriptions.

The details of my work locations, and the hospitals where I was treated, are composite descriptions from a variety of settings. Each work or treatment site is, therefore, a fictional place for the purpose of telling my story. Each individual, other than those who are specifically named with their permission, is fictitious. The fictional names and descriptions are assigned to various characters for the purpose of telling the story from my perspective. I, however, am a completely real character in my story, and the experiences and lessons are how I remember them.

My Gaucher Disease narrative begins before a treatment existed, and extends well beyond. I picked up a few experiences, many friends, and a few lessons that will always affect me personally and professionally. This is my story of a life with Gaucher Disease.

Wayne Rosenfield
Parrish, Florida
June 14, 2015

1.

"Sign here. You're going to inpatient psych."

In the darkened room, I knew my patient could hear me even though her eyes were closed. Lying on a low bed with protective rails all around her, she lifted her right hand and I put a pen into it. She signed the Request for Voluntary Admission to Psychiatric Treatment, a standard statewide form. There are places for some demographic information on the top third of the page. The rest of the sheet has a lot of fine print, quoting the state statutes that apply to inpatient psychiatric hospitalization. Here, in the Emergency Department, conversations tend to be short. It's not the place for psychotherapy. A psychologist in this environment needs to form a relationship with a patient quickly, and then conduct a very focused interview. But I already knew this patient from a prior admission. I remembered very well that I had seen her tearfully depressed in the past, in an episode that lasted for weeks. There are people who truly suffer with their mental disorders, and she is one of them. It is hard for me to fully appreciate the conditions that she must be enduring, to have reached a conclusion that hers is not a life that is worth living.

In the hours prior to this encounter in the Emergency Department, she did, once again, come to that conclusion. She swallowed all of her psychiatric medications, with the knowledge that one of them is dangerous at high doses. She knew that the amount of medication available to her was probably enough to cause her to die. This was a suicide attempt by means of drug overdose.

I have always used the word charcoal as a noun, something we use at barbecues. In the Emergency Department, charcoal is a verb. A patient may be "charcoaled" at the suggestion of Poison Control. The patient would have arrived in the Emergency Department by ambulance, comfortably tucked into a rolling gurney with the scissor-like legs, a warm blanket covering her, a restraining belt around her abdomen, a heart monitor taking up some free space next to her, and an oxygen mask over her face. The emergency medical technicians riding with her in the ambulance would have contacted the Emergency Department by radio while inbound, so that communication with the nurses would not waste precious seconds upon arrival. Once inside the hospital, the nurses would have immediately evaluated her pulse, respiration, and blood pressure. They would have obtained as much information as possible about the circumstances and events preceding arrival. Then the nurses would have informed the emergency physician regarding the patient's condition. The physician would direct the treatment, trying to ensure the patient's survival.

This is where charcoal transforms from a noun to a verb. Life on Earth is based on the chemistry of carbon. And, in this circumstance, a carbon compound is used to absorb the chemicals that endanger a person's life. I have seen many people come into Emergency Departments following drug overdoses, some motivated by suicidal intent and some whose ingestions were accidental, or just ill advised. I don't know the details of the medical and nursing treatments. Really, I just know what I have seen the nurses and physicians doing from a distance.

I also don't know what happens to all of that charcoal when it finishes traversing the patient's digestive system. I did see what happened the next day after our dog ate some mouse poison and was charcoaled by the veterinarian. It can't be pleasant.

The psychologist in the Emergency Department is involved after the patient is declared to be "medically cleared." It's no longer a medical emergency at that point, and the person is considered to be physically healthy. But, there is always a lot more to the story. This patient, previously known to me, had reached a conclusion, on this day, that her very consciousness was too painful a burden. Now it is time for the psychologist to act, to figure out where this is coming from and what to do about it. Of course she needed to be in the hospital. The disposition of a case such as this is not a hard decision.

This being a job, two days later I needed to fill out my timesheet. I went upstairs to the inpatient psychiatric unit. This is a discretely labeled door that cannot be readily opened. I do get a certain feeling of satisfaction from swiping my badge over the sensor and hearing the door unlock. It is similar to the feeling upon entering the Emergency Department, swiping the badge and seeing the door labeled "Authorized Personnel Only" swing open for me. I must be important. All those years of classes and papers and collection of research data have come to this: I can make doors open.

I hadn't yet reached the office where I would find my timesheet; I was still walking through the large, comfortable living room with soft chairs and couches. It's a quiet place that is physically comfortable and inviting. I'm reminded that, in past years, a place such as this was called an asylum. We can do much more now than simply provide a place of refuge from a painful world. We think we can change some of the social, behavioral, family, emotional, and even neurochemical conditions that lead people to conclude that their lives are not worth living. It's very hard for me to fully conceive of the depth of the pain, the hopelessness, and the utter psychological desolation that would lead a person to this place. But I do know how to recognize it. I know, well at least I think I know, what to do about it.

On this day, as I walked through this environment with a specific task in mind — oh yes, it's timesheet day — I saw my patient from the Emergency Department earlier in the week. She watched me as I crossed the room, with a puzzled look on her face. I didn't see anger or anguish, but certainly not happiness either. I detoured around a large, low chair with a heavy wooden frame. The furniture is like what I remember from college dormitories: heavy and durable. The furniture seems to be intended for much use, and cannot be easily thrown. I approached the young woman, now fully awake and responsive, well past the effects of her drug overdose. "Do you remember me?" I asked her. I didn't know at that time how she might be feeling about being there, or how she might be feeling about me, from the perspective of being inside a unit with a locked door. I recalled the young man I saw in an Emergency Department years earlier who awoke following his drug overdose and, seeing me standing over him, was most unhappy to discover that he was still alive. On this occasion, this woman in the locked unit sitting on the durable furniture asked, "Are you the person I saw in the Emergency Department who got me up here?"
"Yes," I answered.
She looked directly into my eyes and said softly, "Thank you."

I don't even remember if I said, "You're welcome" or some other self-important platitude. What I do remember is the thought, "How did I get here? How did I get to be the person who can properly evaluate an emergency condition and be in the right place with the right credentials and knowledge and emotional fortitude to voluntarily work in a setting such as this, and to know what to do to help people?" It's not about having a badge showing a big, red "PhD" that I can wave like a sorcerer's wand and make a door that says, "Authorized Personnel Only" swing open. It's about being the right person, at the right time and place, willing to be immersed within extraordinarily intense situations, and to be capable and motivated to do the right things. How does that happen?

2.

My thoughts turned to the very beginnings of my interest in science. I recalled having several childhood diseases in rapid succession during my kindergarten year. There were no vaccines in those days for measles, mumps, or chicken pox. I had rubella too, but that was six years later. My parents dutifully brought me to the pediatrician. But there was no treatment that I can remember, except to put a soothing lotion on the itchy eruptions.

Everyone got these diseases. I didn't know anyone personally who had a major problem with one of them. These were rites of passage. My classmates spoke of other rites of passage, such as going with Grandma to buy a cute, white dress for First Communion, or with Dad to buy a catcher's mitt. I had neither of those. Nobody dreamed of putting me into a dress and I can't think of anyone in my family who knew what to do with a catcher's mitt. One of my rites was to attend incomprehensible and never-ending services in the synagogue, in the fall, at the time of year when school started on days with chilly mornings, when the maple trees had a touch of red.

The pediatrician remarked to my parents that I had a large spleen. "He has a large spleen," he said. "Some children have large spleens." And with this statement a crucial empirical observation was summarily dismissed. And I also had frequent nosebleeds. "Hold his head back," came the sage advice. And I was fatigued. And the blood chemistries showed something unusual, although I don't know what it was. "He has infectious mononucleosis," my parents were told. "That's the kissing disease. Who have you been kissing, young man?"

I must have mumbled something, but it was surely unremarkable or my parents would have repeated it back to me for decades. They thought I was a prodigy of some sort. My grandfather said that I made more sense than the old men he knew from synagogue. And a *shohet* in my grandfather's poultry business, a Lubavitcher Hasidic rabbi, asked my father to enroll me in his *yeshiva*. "I'll make him a scholar," he said. A *shohet* is the person entrusted to kill animals in the manner that will make them kosher. And enrollment in a *yeshiva* would mean some intense religious training and a very different course to my life. My Hebrew would have been a lot better. But no, I was going to kindergarten in a public school.

I was at home with my mother because I was sick. We watched television together. We watched grainy, black and white television together. I recall the children's shows, some of which are now immortal, and some that were hokey, local productions. I don't remember watching any news programs, but I surely did. When I returned to school, my kindergarten teacher remarked to my mother that I knew all about *Sputnik*, which had been launched a year earlier, and I was the only pupil (we were called pupils in Massachusetts) who knew what was currently going on in the world. My world's horizon was beyond sitting on the floor, cross-legged, in front of a nurturing kindergarten teacher.

The following year included more exposure to the news, especially because someone from our state was running for President. I learned to read that year, English and Hebrew. During the next year my class walked together ("Slow down. Hold hands.") to a nearby branch library for some sort of very forgettable story time. On the way to the library I noticed that many people were lining the street, as if for a parade. My ability to read must have been adequate by that time because I remember that one of the people on a second floor porch was holding a sign that said, "Welcome back, Jack." Inside the library we listened to the exploits of, I don't know, probably some talking farm animal, but I really wanted to be outside on the street. The droning monotone of the librarian's voice was interrupted by a huge roar from the crowd outside, which quickly subsided. And that's how I missed seeing our Senator John Kennedy while he campaigned to be President.

*

Standing before my depressed, recently suicidal and now thankful patient, I recalled all these things, without a lucid answer to my question about how my life's path brought me to this spot, to be the right person at the right time, positioned to do the right things. Then I recalled my third grade teacher, who saw my interest in science and tried to encourage it. I noticed at the time that I seemed to get called upon for an answer more than my classmates. And I was the only pupil (welcome to Massachusetts) who did a science demonstration in front of the class. It was just a small volcano, but I was the only student to do it.

I know as a scientist, and also because Albert Einstein said it earlier that every great result is built upon the work of others. When I walked across the stage at the Jorgensen Auditorium on the campus of the University of Connecticut, to be handed a diploma, to be turned toward the audience by two professors who then dressed me in the hood of my degree, repositioned my hat, and directed me to the president of the university who shook my hand with a "congratulations, doctor," my honor was partially owned by many people whom I encountered earlier.

My third grade teacher was the first to nurture my interest in science, and she is a part owner of whatever I accomplish. Not too many years ago I found her. It was important to me to inform her of the reach of her work.

3.

Not every year of my life has specific memories to distinguish it from other years. The indistinguishable years seem to increase in frequency with advancing years. And it's not just a matter of forgetfulness. There are years of great change or growth. And there are years distinguished by some life event. But at some point, there is a certain routine in effect that causes years to slide seamlessly into each other.

Fourth grade was distinguished by my grandmother's cardiac problems while she and my grandfather were spending their usual winter in Miami Beach. For people who came to New England from Eastern Europe, they were pretty intolerant of snow. My Mom's absence while she was in Florida taking care of her parents was more traumatic than the daily drills of multiplication tables and my struggle with long division. An assignment to memorize Longfellow's "Paul Revere's Ride" was the only blatant indoctrination to Massachusetts culture. We were also taught that the pilgrims in Plymouth were the first Europeans to settle in North America. Only later did I learn, independent of my Massachusetts education that the pilgrims in Plymouth had actually been trying to reach the existing settlement at Jamestown. I now know to be skeptical of what I'm taught.

Fifth grade snuck up on me, and I have no idea why I was grouped with pupils (yes, pupils) who were advanced in math. It was not until my doctoral program that I fully realized how different Longfellow's achievements are from Euclid's. They are separated by a vast crevice in my head, called the central commissure, and there is a narrow connection between them, called the *corpus callosum*. I could not have imagined that fatigue, a large spleen, a diagnosis (or maybe it was an accusation) of infectious mononucleosis, and nosebleeds, could all be related, and may even have some connection with my early struggles with math. It's not that I couldn't learn the math. It's just that the spatial and numeric relationships were not as intuitively easy for me as verbal abstraction, memory, and communication.

I could not have imagined that all of these disparate observations were connected. Nor could I have foreseen what would happen next. I lived nine-tenths of a mile from my school. School bus transportation, and the privilege of eating lunch in the building, were reserved only for students who lived at a distance of one mile or more. It was a pleasant walk to school in the morning, home for lunch, back to school, and then home again in the afternoon, walking past the Shriners Hospital for Crippled Children four times each day. Are any current students required to walk more than three and a half miles per day just to attend school and have lunch? Let me resist the digression into social commentary about narcissism in our sedentary culture. (Sorry, I couldn't help it.)

On one of these days about a month into the school year, my right leg hurt when I returned home in the afternoon. The pain wasn't too bad, but my thigh ached. And rather than abating, the pain seemed to become sharper, even stabbing. And the pain continued to intensify. I told my Mom who was, of course, properly concerned. I could not sleep that night, and my Mom sat up with me. There is nothing on Earth like a parent's love and, especially, maternal protectiveness. In college I saw it in the eyes of the research animals when I was involved with breeding the next semester's rats. I saw it many times from my mother, and I saw it also from my wife.

Again consulting the pediatrician, my parents were told that I probably had a muscle strain of some sort. Day after day I endured intractable pain. There was no relief. And there was no explanation. At night, sitting on my father's reclining chair in the living room, I remember tearfully apologizing to my Mom. I could see the agony on her face as I cried until exhaustion knocked me out for a few hours. The pediatrician instructed my parents to bring me to the hospital, where my leg was x-rayed. Still there was no explanation for my pain. I was admitted to the inpatient pediatric ward. Laboratory tests seemed to suggest an infection, or maybe it was leukemia. There was a brief suggestion that I was a whining, complaining sort of kid. In the hospital I received my first medication for pain. Whether I was improving as a result of the pain medication, I don't know. But the pain was becoming more tolerable.

I shared a room with three other children. My roommates included a boy younger than I was, named Donny. He had the loudest voice of any of us, which we frequently exploited to call the nurses. Donny also had hemophilia. His mother came to visit him every day. I can only imagine how Donny's mother's heart must have ached for him. Even then, hemophilia was known to be a genetic disorder passed from mothers to sons. In the morning, when the lady with the needles came for Donny's blood, he needed a pile of pads for the bleeding that followed.

At play therapy during the day, in the playroom at the end of the hall, I met a girl a couple of years older than me. She laughed that she was there because she could not stop her hiccups. Not being able to stop the hiccups sounded very inconvenient to me. In the days that followed I learned that her hiccups were related to a brain tumor. The last time I saw her, she was lying on a stretcher, apparently sedated, with her head wrapped in white bandages. I don't know where she was going, and I don't know what became of her. Neither do I know what became of Donny, although I am aware that most of a generation of men with hemophilia died from a contaminated infusion product that was supposed to save their lives.

My doctor ordered ever more invasive tests. I had a "spinal tap." It hurt. Then I had a bone marrow biopsy. I didn't see the needle that the pediatric resident was leaning into, almost turning me over with the force. That hurt too. Then I had a lymph node biopsy taken from my groin, which was the first time that I saw the inside of an operating room. My leg was numb with a local anesthetic and I remember the kindness of the surgical nurse who asked the surgeon if I could suck on an ice cube. The surgeon consented, and he also showed me the tissue he had extracted, grasped on the end of a shiny instrument.

Back in my room, three weeks into this ordeal, I was feeling better. I received a packet of get-well cards from my classmates. The pediatrician told my parents that I probably had endured an infection of some sort. He called it osteomyelitis. When my father questioned him further about how all of this could happen, and how to prevent a recurrence, the pediatrician dismissed him with "He's getting better, isn't he?" My father asked him if there could be a specialist somewhere who could provide a better explanation for what had happened to me. The answer given to my Dad was, "When someone wants a second opinion, they call me." The diagnostic dots had not been connected, and the professional had dismissed his own empirical observations, as well as the concerns of the parent. When future events and other professionals added to the body of information, my father let the pediatrician know that he had missed something big. And my Dad never forgave him.

*

My painful October, early in fifth grade, was the last full month of the Kennedy presidency, a time in American history sometimes referred to as Camelot. By late November I was again walking both ways to school. Just down the street from my elementary school I would pass a huge, ornate Catholic church. And then I would cross the street at a big intersection presided-over by a policeman, who would give us a hand sign when it was safe to cross. A few more steps and I would be near a tiny fish market with a fan over the door. On Fridays the fan blew the smell of fried fish into the street. It smelled absolutely delicious.

On Friday, November the twenty-second, the church's bells were pealing in the afternoon. I have no memory of the smell of fried fish on that day. This was Massachusetts, one of our own was President, and he had just been murdered.

*

The next few years were again of the seamlessly sliding variety. I was once again in a math class beyond my comprehension. From my current perspective, finding the prime factors of an integer is not a problem. But at that time it was a mystery. MAD Magazine corrupted me, and I especially liked the "Snappy Answers to Foolish Questions." In recent years, a cardiologist at a prestigious medical center, assessing me to rule out increased blood pressure in my pulmonary artery, a condition for which I have a slightly increased risk, performed an echocardiogram with Doppler measurement of the tricuspid regurgitation. When it was over he asked me if I had any questions. "Yes," I said. "What are the prime factors of forty-one?"

My grandfather, my last surviving grandparent, died four months before I became a *Bar Mitzvah*. I learned much more about him in the following years. I had especially liked his jokes and his wry view of everyday life. Many years later I was able to access historical records involving Minsk, his hometown. And I discovered why his family's fate during the Holocaust was never spoken of. I now think that his humor hid a broken heart. My older son is named for him.

4.

The next year, again in September, I had another episode of searing pain in my right thigh. My parents took me to an orthopaedic surgeon. The suggestion was that I had a muscle inflammation. He called it "synovitis." The condition resolved fairly quickly, probably within two weeks, as best as I can remember.

The following year, again in September, my hip was painful. Walking was a chore. I pressed on, until one day, arriving at home after school, I could barely move. I dragged myself onto my bed. I told my parents that something was very wrong. I asked them to call the orthopaedist again, because the leg felt the way it had a year earlier. We lived less than a mile from the community hospital. The orthopaedic surgeon stopped by to see me in the evening, on his way home from his rounds in the hospital.

The next day my right hip and thigh were x-rayed. My father spoke to the orthopaedist and the report I heard was "there are dramatic changes" in the hip. I learned the details later, that my right femoral head had a massive avascular necrosis, and was partially collapsed. In plain language, the round part of my thighbone that is the ball part of the hip joint was no longer living bone. It had lost the structural strength to hold me, and it had crushed under my weight.

I was admitted to the hospital, pediatrics again, for tests. Our family doctor, whose specialty happened to be hematology, saw me in the hospital. He repeated the bone marrow biopsy that I had found so distasteful five years earlier. I must say, he was much better at it than the pediatric resident. And he reexamined the earlier results, including the lymph node biopsy. My history was full of important clues. I had a large spleen. I had a tendency to be anemic. My platelets were low. I had suffered an avascular necrosis of the hip. There were some other laboratory observations which could indicate leukemia, or mononucleosis, although those illnesses were not consistent with the overall picture.

Years later, when I studied research design, I learned that a good theory is the most parsimonious explanation for all of the data. Only one valid datum that is not explained by a theory is sufficient to invalidate the theory. And a scientist of integrity cannot reject data that do not support his theory. Data represent reality. A theory is just our attempt to explain our observations simply. A good theory incorporates all known information, and attempts to explain it. All of the clues were there. What I needed was a scientist to connect them into a single explanatory theory.

My doctor was also very aware that we are a Jewish family of Eastern European descent. We are from a subgroup of Jews known as Ashkenazi. To historians that means that we are descendants of the Jewish group whose western migration was to the area of Germany known as *Ashkenaz*. To me it meant that a certain letter in the Hebrew alphabet was to be pronounced with an "S" sound instead of a "T". But most relevant to me, being Ashkenazi meant that our food was at times greasy, and included pickled herring, boiled potatoes with sour cream, borscht, matzoh balls and noodle casserole; all of which were menu items brought from Eastern Europe. We also had bagels, which our people invented in New York, and we put cream cheese and smoked salmon on them, which would have been way too extravagant a delicacy in Russia. And we were a pickling sort of people, which we demonstrated with cucumbers, tomatoes, cabbage, beets, and corned beef brisket. There were many people from our group with recognizable names, such as Kafka, Freud, and Einstein. There was a resort region in the Catskill Mountains known colloquially as the Borscht Belt. We had our favorites on television too, people with normal, American sounding names like Tony Curtis and Jack Benny. But we knew that underneath the stage names were people from our own tribe. It was a fact that we called Saturday *Shabbos* and not *Shabbat*. It was a fact that the vast majority of Jews in the United States were Ashkenazi. And it was also a fact that the Jews of Eastern Europe had been segregated from the surrounding populations for perhaps fifteen centuries, plus or minus a few generations.

There is a concentration of certain genetic characteristics in this population. It would be more accurate to say that this inbred group has a concentration of certain mutations. But in 1968, in this pediatric ward in Massachusetts, we were not sufficiently sophisticated to speak of mutations. My doctor knew how bone marrow was supposed to appear under his microscope. And he surely knew that he was seeing something abnormal. In the eye of a scientist observing important clues, and possessing the knowledge to interpret his observations within an empirical framework, the diagnosis was clear. His report to my parents was confident and authoritative. "Wayne has Gaucher's Disease," he said.

5.

I was informed later of this diagnosis, although the information had no practical meaning. The name of this illness was the total of what we knew about it. The diagnosis meant nothing to us. When we discussed it, my parents each looked vaguely downward, their faces expressionless and without movement. We were all now aware of the diagnosis, but no one knew enough to even ask the next question. "How did he catch Gaucher's Disease?" my mother wondered aloud.

Additional snippets of information entered the conversation in the coming days. This was somehow connected to us being Jewish. I was still in the hospital, during a visit by our rabbi, when my father shared this part of the overall picture. The rabbi was visibly shaken by this revelation. The news that being Jewish is somehow related to being seriously physically messed up is, well, a little difficult to absorb.

My parents were also told that a child with Gaucher's Disease has parents who both carry it, and that is how the child got sick. When my Dad was driving lawfully on the Massachusetts Turnpike, well below the speed limit, and he saw a policeman, he slowed down. So I knew that he felt guilty even in the best of times. But this... His prodigal son, his firstborn, was hurt. And the message that he took away from conversations with the doctor was that he, the father who wanted more than anything to protect his child, was implicated in the child's injury. My Dad often said that his life began when he met his

Muriel. And now he thought of how selfish he must be, married to someone who makes him happy, whose marriage has hurt their son.

*

My Dad often told me that he would have preferred to be stricken in some way himself, if the misfortune could have been deflected from me. I accepted that statement at the time as a loving sentiment. But I have come to realize since then that the love a parent feels for a child is genuine altruism. I had already seen my mother's devotion to her children. Years later, when I visited my Mom every week in the nursing home, her muscles frozen by Parkinson's Disease, I reminded her of those nights when she sat with me when I needed her most. And I told her that she had earned the devotion of her son.

In college, when I reached into a cage to pick up a rat pup, the mommy rat, descended from thousands of generations of animals bred for their docility and friendliness to undergraduates, slowly circled my hand. The look in her eye said, "Back off and close the cage," which I did. The mommy rat was a vegetarian and not predatory toward psychology students. But she had some huge front teeth and a primal protectiveness of her offspring. Years later, when an elementary school teacher was destructively critical of my older son, I saw that same look in the eye of his mother, my wife. And when the parent-teacher conference was done, the point had been made. Whether this was the reason that the teacher left town at the end of the academic year, I don't know. But at the time, I said to my wife, "I know that look. Those are lioness behaviors. I saw it in National Geographic."

The parents' intense protectiveness of their children is so cruelly exploited by the circumstances of a genetic disorder. The very circumstances that gave life to the child, also gave the disorder. And so, my parents' guilt was intense and they felt personally responsible for everything that was happening to me.

6.

I suggested to my father that we should go to the library to see what we could learn about Gaucher's Disease. The public library in my hometown is a huge building of white marble, with Corinthian columns. On the lawn stands a large bronze statue of one of the Puritans who governed at the time of the settlement's founding in 1636. He was a scary looking guy.

The inside of the library was a quiet place that smelled like dust. We found a medical dictionary and brought it to one of the long tables made of a dark wood. My Dad put his hand on the volume and looked directly at me. "Are you sure you want to open it?" he asked. I wasn't sure that I knew what he was nervous about. I found the entry on Gaucher's Disease and saw impossible words such as *hepatosplenamegaly* and *thrombocytopenia* and *glucocerebrosidase*. There was some indication, as I recall, that this disorder is very unusual and can be related to cognitive problems. I didn't feel informed by what I read, but at least I had the name for the problem.

The orthopaedic surgeon who was involved with this turn of events that now had a name, had heard of Gaucher's Disease. He said that he attended a lecture about it when he was in medical school in New York. He said the lecture was given by an orthopaedic surgeon in New York who seemed to know a lot about Gaucher's Disease. The doctor in New York was doing "a study" of some sort. "Maybe," my orthopaedist in Massachusetts told us, "he'll see Wayne."

*

My father got the contact information for the New York doctor and I was informed that we had an appointment. This was the third time that I had experienced an episode of a painful leg, so I expected that this would all be resolved in a few weeks, just as before. For now, however, I would be walking on crutches, without putting any weight on the leg.

My parents brought me, on one sunny, but cool, autumn day, to New York. This was a neighborhood that my father told me was not safe and he instructed me to stay close to them. I was not a fan of my father's over protectiveness and while he did whatever he needed to do with the car, I walked ahead, on my crutches, and went into the building. I don't recall if there was a valet for the car, but I think so. My father was quite panicked when he turned around and didn't see me. The day was already charged with emotion as we found the elevator and located the Orthopaedics Department.

My father was notably calmer when he met the doctor. The name of my new doctor was Henry J. Mankin, MD. He appeared to be about the same age as my parents, which was relatively young to be a medical school professor. My Dad was a salesman, and he had a way of striking up a conversation with almost anyone. At this first encounter with my new doctor I would expect that my Dad assessed what he had in common with his conversation partner, looking first for a Masonic ring and, failing that, by throwing a few words of Yiddish into the conversation. Jackpot! The doctor who can help Wayne with this Gaucher's Disease thing is Jewish. My new doctor was animated, energetic, and talkative. He asked me what had happened to me. Dr. Mankin answered simply, "I know the story well."

*

I had a complete skeletal survey that day, x-rays of all of my bones. I still had two hundred and six of them, although one of them was in trouble. At the end of the day I was advised that I would need to stay off of my hip. I would need to maintain a condition of "non-weight-bearing." This would allow the area of necrosis to revascularize without further damage. After the bone is revascularized, I could then have surgery to fix the damage that had occurred. So far, so good. I was still on board with this plan.

"How long will I need to use crutches?" I asked.
"It will take about three years," came the words from the expert.

He might as well have punched me in the head. I felt panicked. This was not in my plans. Next year I would be old enough to take driving lessons, and I had a full agenda of teenager things that I would rather be doing.

On the drive home from New York, my parents were exuberant. They had an animated conversation in the front seat while there was nothing but gloom in back with me. Three years! This Jewish doctor must not be much of an expert if I would be spending my high school years walking with crutches. But Dr. Mankin would eventually become my hero, and my parents were grateful to him for the rest of their lives.

7.

I think I moped around the house for about three days. Life was empty and meaningless. In cognitive therapy we try to discern the "internal dialogue." I cannot say what I was thinking at the time. But somehow I got the notion that, if I'm going to be using my arms for locomotion, I'd better strengthen them.

My parents seemed willing to provide me with a membership at a gym. I was the only person in the weight room who arrived on crutches. My goal was to bench press my own weight. That seemed logically to be what I needed to do, if I would be carrying myself with my arms. I also did pull-ups on the horizontal bar and I could flip myself all the way around it. I held on tight, never falling, and always keeping my legs off the floor. The one mental statement I remember saying to myself at the time was "If I need to walk on crutches, I'm going to be the best at it that anyone has ever seen." Some of the older men in the gym seemed concerned that I was going to hurt myself. One of them stood close by while I was on the horizontal bar, apparently ready to catch me if necessary. Another one encouraged my bench press sets and was a willing spotter.

I had friends in the neighborhood that sometimes went to the gym with me. But mostly we played with radios and even managed to transmit a signal across the street. This was not the amateur radio that I did for real, many years later. We had small handheld radios with a range slightly greater than the distance we could shout. I had a shortwave receiver that occupied many nighttime hours. I would listen to the government broadcasts from dozens of countries. I had a microscope too, and I sometimes immersed myself in that otherwise invisible world. I learned about photography, but not the aesthetic art of producing great pictures. I taught myself the chemical processes that were necessary after opening the roll of film in the dark. I make no pretense of understanding the chemistry. I had some black and white photographs to show for the effort. I built some model rockets, which never got off the ground.*

I thought that fermenting some grape juice would be an interesting project. I did produce a drinkable wine. I got the idea that, if I put my fermenting brew into an empty champagne bottle and hammered a cork into the top, I would get a sparkling wine. It was a nice try. I achieved more propulsion for that cork than I did for my rocket. I'm just glad that I wasn't in my room when the cork started ricocheting in all directions. I had no well-developed competency in any of these things. I just liked to dabble, to follow my curiosity. If I were ever shipwrecked, I think that I could likely make a signaling device, or maybe even some wine, before I would ever figure out how to fix the boat.

I cannot say that I was coping entirely well. I was embarrassed to go to school with crutches and I prevailed upon my parents to ask for a teacher to come to the house. The school system did provide a homebound teacher for a couple of months.

---

*I did have a successful launch years later, with my sons. The solid propellant sent the tiny projectile up hundreds of feet, the parachute deployed, and that was the last we ever saw of my rocket.

But then, somewhere in the public school bureaucracy, in a building across the street from the library and the scary Puritan, a person whom I never knew decided at some point that I belonged in school and not at home. High school at home was coming to an end. I resented this intrusion upon my independent choice. I was fifteen years old and still knew everything.

8.

I reentered high school, a huge multi-floored building constructed in 1898. Built prior to widespread availability of electric lights, it was designed around many courtyards, so that interior rooms would get sunlight. It was not designed for accessibility by someone using crutches. But I was in great physical condition, the avascular necrosis notwithstanding. I ignored my mobility issues. I walked home from school, about three and one-half miles. I moved very quickly, even with books tucked between my left arm and the crutch.

I carried my trumpet case too, until my parents brought me for a non-medical trip to New York to buy a really good horn. The carrying case for a King Super 20 was too big to carry with crutches. It was well known in the brass section that I had a King. The word on the street was that our idol, Doc Severinsen on The Tonight Show, played a King Silver Flair. I was in the band, jazz band, and orchestra playing trumpet, second chair. And while I was no Doc Severinsen, I was elected to be band vice president.

My high school instrumental music teacher, the conductor for all of these groups, walked with a limp. He was genuinely empathic to me and seemed to understand my predicament. He revealed to me that he had survived polio as a child. At several times during the school year our various ensembles would perform as a community service. One such gig — we musicians refer to our performances as gigs — was due to be at the Shriners Hospital for Crippled Children, the building near my home that I had passed walking to and from my elementary school. In later years, when polio was no longer a scourge of childhood, the facility was renamed simply as Shriners Hospital.

This hospital was in my neighborhood, but I had never been inside. Our music teacher felt the need to say a few words of preparation to his young musicians prior to the gig. He was brief in his remarks. "You're going to see a lot of children in various stages of disrepair." I knew that he was understating his feeling for these children.

Inside the Shriners Hospital for Crippled Children we saw children with all manner of mobility problems. We performed the pieces that we had rehearsed, but we did not interact personally with any of the young patients. Our worlds were profoundly different. I felt that I understood their world, but I could not bear to get closer to it.

I survived some advanced math courses and I hoped that I would never again see the formula for the slope of a line. Of what practical use is that foolish $y=mx+b$ equation and why would I ever need to know it? That question awaited an answer.

*

My parents brought me to see Dr. Mankin every three months. The appointments had a predictable routine. I would first have x-rays of my hip. I would bring the films from the Radiology Department to the doctor's office. Inside the examination room the doctor would take the films from the large envelope and put them on a light board. He would point to the area of my femoral head that was showing new bone growth. Dr. Mankin would say something positive and conclude with "I'll see you in three months." That was the pattern for over two years.

The summer before my senior year of high school included some visits to possible colleges. I was ready to get out of town. I settled upon Alfred University, a small, private university in a very rural area, about ninety miles from Buffalo. I received an early acceptance to Alfred University, about seven months prior to high school graduation. My hip was becoming as healed as it would ever be without some surgical help. The plan was to have the hip reconstruction surgery shortly after graduation.

As the school year ended, graduating seniors received various academic honors. I recall hearing a murmur from my assembled classmates as I walked with a painful limp across the stage to receive an award for writing. It was the first academic award that I ever received for anything. And it was the first time that most of them had ever seen me move without crutches. I had the appearance and the expectation of great improvement in my condition. But there is a Yiddish proverb that says, *"Mensch tracht und Gott lacht,"* "Man plans and God laughs." This was very nearly the last month of my life.

9.

Two weeks after graduation from high school my parents drove me to the hospital in New York. I was one of four young men in a rectangular room. There was a window behind me, near my bed. The only direct sunlight was in the late afternoon.

I was admitted three days prior to my planned surgery, for "tests." Various physicians came to see me, and did weird things to me. One of them made my ear bleed. Another one of them put a blood pressure cuff on my arm and pumped it up. Then he seemed to be keeping track of the time while my hand turned an unnatural color. I still didn't know what *thrombocytopenia* meant. But someone else certainly did, and the issue got a lot of attention.

On the day of surgery I watched the ceiling tiles along the way to the surgical suite. I went through several doorways and, after passing the last one, the room smelled funny, like rubber. I don't know why it smelled like that. But the smell meant to me that I was in a place outside of normal experience. I felt very cold. Someone put a warm blanket over me, and my conscious awareness ended.

*

My next awareness was of being in a nightmare from which I could not awaken. I could not move. I was nauseous. My ankles were bound to a wooden pole, an "abduction bar," I would later learn. I cannot say how much time passed before I was again in my room. But the pain in my hip was searing. Dr. Mankin appeared at my bedside and I asked him when I could go home. "When it's time," he said, without even a trace of a smile. I told my parents that he was grouchy.

I looked forward to the injections of a narcotic every four hours. The nurses were mean and uncaring. On one occasion when I called for the nurse so I could have my pain medication, she leaned on the doorframe at the entrance to the room with her arms crossed and impatiently asked me, "What's the emergency?"

The next morning some of my blood was drawn by an emissary from the laboratory. I was also receiving blood through an intravenous line, and I watched it drip with its steady rhythm. My awareness of time was distorted. Later that day, or maybe it was the next day, or the day after that, an orthopaedic resident came to my bed. He grabbed the sheet covering me and pulled it off. He looked me over from head to toe. He checked the sheet under me. He seemed to be looking for something. He remarked that my leg was very swollen. He revealed that the laboratory results showed that I was bleeding. Actually he said, "You are bleeding quite a lot." The only question was, "Where is the blood?"

The conclusion was that I was bleeding into the leg. But there was more to the story. The reason for Dr. Mankin's serious face days earlier, immediately after surgery, was that he was very, very worried about me. My bleeding started during the surgery. He surely worked quickly and deliberately to normalize the shape of my femoral head, to give me what he called "a usable hip." During the surgery, donor blood was going into my arm at a rate slightly less than the rate at which blood was coming out of the wound. The total quantity of transfused blood was more than my normal blood volume. I had bled out and was alive only because of the availability of donor blood. Years later, Dr. Mankin would introduce me to some orthopaedic residents saying, "This is Wayne. Following surgery he bled into the wound and I bled into my gut." He told me privately, "You almost died."

*

Later in the week I was able to dangle my feet over the bed. And when the abduction bar was removed and I could get out of the bed, one of the few compassionate nurses wheeled me to the toilet. Using a toilet would be a milestone, my re-entry into normal life. The nurse waited outside the door and I am grateful for that. I managed to squeak out some sort of distress call and she rushed in to catch me before I fell on the floor. I did not have the energy to remain vertical for long.

Finally the day arrived when my parents could come from Massachusetts to bring me home. I watched the street from the window next to my bed and I was thrilled to see the familiar car and my rescuers, a half dozen floors below. For the trip they brought my girlfriend too, which completed my sense of returning to a normal life. I had lost quite a lot of weight. But I have always had a healthy appetite and I was happy to obey the order to eat. I was getting around on crutches initially. Some time during the summer I began to use a cane.

10.

I was still using a cane when, in September, my parents drove me to Alfred University. I would be a student in a part of the world, which, even today, is known as The Niagara Frontier. This rural area southeast of Buffalo is known for bitingly cold winters with prodigious amounts of snow. My parents exhibited a great deal of courage in leaving me at this university, far from home, so soon after the surgery experience.

I was aware of a liberal arts graduation requirement for two courses in either physical education or military science. I thought, at the time, that there were no realistic physical education courses for me. But military science sounded oh-so-interesting. I envisioned learning about the tactics and circumstances of great battles in history.

I arrived for the morning class and, after signing something and taking an oath to defend the US Constitution, I finally realized that I had just joined Army ROTC. After a long lecture by an upperclassman about how to shine my buttons, how my hair was to be cut, and the importance of straight lines while marching, I found the office of my commanding officer. He was a US Army colonel who had earlier in the day introduced himself and reported that he had just recently returned from yet another combat tour in Vietnam. He was very understanding when I said, "This isn't for me" and that I would be dropping the course. Before the day ended I was enrolled in trumpet lessons in the Performing Arts Department. My military career had lasted less than six hours.

*

By November of my first semester, my gait stability and pain level enabled me to put away the cane. I still had a limited walking range before the pain increased. But I was quite pleased that I had achieved a new normal.

My grades that first year were acceptable but not remarkable. The following September, at the start of sophomore year, I found the chairman of the Psychology Department and I told him that I was thinking of majoring in psychology. I told him that I envisioned a career as a psychologist. His answer, "Best move you'll ever make," was supportive and welcoming, and more prophetic than he would ever know.

"That's nice," my father noted approvingly, "but can you make a living with that?" I told him that this would be a very competitive field, and that I would be successful only if I could be among the best. I was on the Dean's List every semester after that.

*

At some point during sophomore year I visited Dr. Mankin, my doctor in New York, with my parents. He seemed to be very serious. He revealed that he had some news to share, announcing that he would be leaving New York. My father's heart sank. My Dad said that we would follow him wherever he goes. We waited for the bad news about how far we would need to travel to stay with the only Gaucher expert we knew.

My doctor said that he would be moving to… to… I could feel my father's tension. "I'll be moving to Boston," said the Jewish Gaucher expert. My father was an emotionally demonstrative person, but he held himself together and did not break into a dance. This was the best possible outcome. My father was originally from the North Shore, and Boston felt like a hometown. Dr. Mankin seemed relieved that we would be willing to continue with him when, really, to my Dad, he had just agreed to move in with us.

Already involved with trumpet lessons as an elective course, I and my King Super 20 joined the concert band, the brass choir, and the jazz ensemble. My ability to read music is mediocre. But I can make a great sound, I can play loud, and I have good range. After playing fourth chair in the Alfred University Jazz Ensemble as a sophomore, I was playing lead trumpet during my junior and senior years. There were actually two of us covering first chair because it's a physically demanding role. And contrary to what is suggested by the title "first chair," the five people playing trumpet in the twenty-two-piece ensemble do not get chairs.

For the summer prior to my senior year of college, I had been accepted into a program involving work on *Kibbutz Kinneret*, a collective farm in southern Galilee. In fact, this kibbutz is the second oldest in Israel. *Kibbutz Kinneret* was founded by Russian Jews who were enthusiastic Bolsheviks. But they were, after all, still Jews, and so they were not welcome participants in the changes occurring in Mother Russia. But the Czar, who was no fan of the Bolsheviks, also had no love for the Jews. So, during the same time period as my grandparents' arrivals in America, other Jews migrated to the ancestral Jewish homeland, to live their Marxist ideals. Ashkenazi Jews may come from the same geographic region, but they can be communist, or capitalist, or something in between. The menu, however, is usually the same.

I saw our family doctor, the same physician who had diagnosed my Gaucher's Disease six years earlier, for my pre-program physical examination. "You have a varicocele," he impassively observed, "just like your Dad." I asked him what this means. He simply said that this referred to some extra blood vessels and "It can affect sperm production." I filed that information away in my well-developed long-term memory, and spent my summer picking grapes in the Jordan Valley.

*

I learned a lot at Alfred University. I was able to take courses in things that I would never have otherwise known anything about. I learned what it means to be liberally educated. I learned to appreciate modern fiction, which was very much a course in existentialism and how to discern the themes in a narrative. I studied religion from an Episcopalian minister with a doctorate from Hebrew Union College. I incubated the worms that live inside of other worms. I saw spirochete bacteria cork screwing through the water, similar to the bacterium already known to cause syphilis and similar to another spirochete that would eventually be implicated in Lyme Disease. I learned about intracellular organelles such as mitochondria and lysosomes. I learned about the complementary processes of oxidation and reduction and how they work together to make a battery. I learned how to predict a weather satellite's orbit and how to use its output to see above our current snow squall. To satisfy the physical education requirements I took a course in personal fitness where my classmates and I designed and followed individually tailored exercise programs. For my other required physical education course I learned archery. And I learned how to dress warmly and how to drive in snow.

I studied beginning and intermediate Russian where I learned, among other things, that much of my Ashkenazi menu is also a Russian menu. My Russian professor came from the region vacated by my grandparents. He was not Jewish, but he spoke Yiddish, which was enough for the Gestapo to send him to a slave labor camp. I asked him about my grandfather's hometown. He paused, took a deep breath, and said simply, "During the war Minsk was totally destroyed."

But mostly, at Alfred University I learned the fundamentals of the science of psychology. I qualified for *Psi Chi*, the national psychology honor society, during my junior year. As a senior I passed oral examination by the faculty to win Departmental Honors in Psychology. Just prior to graduation I learned that I was also in *Pi Gamma Mu*, the national social science honor society.

During my senior year I already had almost enough credits to graduate. So, during my last semester I was taking only a few courses, mostly related to my interest in all things Russian. I had the luxury of spending much of my time doing things that I enjoyed, such as taking care of laboratory animals, assisting students in the course on operant learning, catching an occasional pass of a weather satellite in the physics department, and playing in the jazz ensemble.

Lining up alphabetically for graduation, my chemistry professor from freshman year was distributing the gold braids that are worn by the graduates whose degrees are granted with honors. As he reached my place in line he did a noticeable double take. I saw him referring again to the graduation program to verify that my name had the asterisk identifying me as an honor graduate. I held out my hand and said softly, "Yeah. That's mine."

11.

I returned to New England to begin graduate school. I had two practicum placements. One was in a residential school for children with severe psychological disorders. The other was in a public school. The world had changed in the five years since I was a public school student, and the presence of a student using a wheelchair to get to class was no longer unusual.

One of my professors invited me to join him for a day of ocean sailing off the coast of Connecticut. With my hand on the tiller I saw a powerboat apparently about to intersect our path. The sailing advice I received was "Just steer a straight course. Let him figure you out." I later recalled this advice as a useful lesson for life.

My fourth year of graduate school had me on the campus of the University of Connecticut as a PhD candidate. My goal to become a psychologist was in sight. The dormitory for the graduate students was a socially unusual place. There were many countries represented, and people were cordial to one another even if not socially involved. Some men from India invited me once to share their spicy rice dish, advising me to be ready with the yogurt because, "It will be difficult for you."

Mostly, doctoral students seemed to be solitary figures, focused and immersed in subjects that no one else would possibly understand. One of my neighbors and I went to a Mexican restaurant one day. His expertise in biochemistry led to a detailed explanation of why the enchiladas produced certain predictable physiological responses. My dictionary defines a nerd as someone who is intelligent but evidencing a single-minded obsession with a nonsocial pursuit. That definition gets no argument from me.

One of the doctoral students in the same dormitory as me was immersed at that time in a discipline far removed from my own. We crossed the same street every day to eat in the same dining hall. Our dissertation defenses were within two months of each other on the same campus, and our degrees were conferred at the same graduation. Our dissertations are one shelf apart in the library. If not for the single-minded absorption of doctoral students, perhaps we would have been friends. We met for the first time, in very recent years, when a pharmaceutical company asked us both, independently, to speak to patient groups about our experiences as people with Gaucher Disease.

I would have liked to speak with some female undergraduates, but I seemed to have very little in common with them. Or maybe they thought that I was a nerd. I was delighted once to be invited to an off-campus party. I think one indicator of the superficiality of the social relationships is that I cannot remember more than a couple of names of the people I encountered at that time.

During the next month after the off-campus party, I found that I didn't feel well. I thought that I might have a fever, but sometimes I felt cold. I thought that maybe I was gaining weight from the college food because my abdomen seemed to be bigger. I was very tired. I took naps in the afternoon, which was unusual for me. Sometimes I felt as though my head was ringing from the inside. At some point I realized that I was having a sharp pain in my left side when taking a deep breath. The campus infirmary was across the street from my advisor's office, so I knew where to find it. And it was *Rosh Hashanah*, the Jewish New Year, so nobody expected me to be working on the various research projects.

I presented myself to the infirmary and, with the precision of a PhD candidate learning empirical methods, I listed my symptoms. During this period the disorder was becoming called *Gaucher* instead of *Gaucher's* and I added that I had been told that I have this diagnosis. I was glad to see the physician's nod, apparently indicating that he was familiar with what I was talking about.

The physician told me that infectious mononucleosis had become quite common on many college campuses this year. My diagnosis on this day truly appeared to be mononucleosis, even after accounting for whatever false indicators were added by the Gaucher Disease. The physician told me that my biggest problem was related to the pain in my left side. He told me that my spleen was huge, and that it was catching on my last rib with each breath. He described the spleen as being like a balloon, and said that mine was quite large and, continuing with the balloon metaphor, "Could pop." I was informed that returning to my dormitory room would not be safe. He said that staying in the infirmary was not a safe option either. The doctor said that I needed to be in a hospital where I could have immediate surgery if it became necessary.

That advice sounded a little alarmist to me, but he seemed to be confident and insistent with his assertion of the danger of the situation. I called my parents who were happy to hear holiday greetings from their son, the almost a doctor. I conveyed the situation to them and the recommendation of the campus physician. Like coaches who have a star player on the bench whom they can put into the game when necessary, my parents said, almost in one voice, that we needed our Gaucher Expert, Dr. Mankin. They drove from their home in western Massachusetts to the University of Connecticut campus, collected me and brought me to Boston.

*

The Emergency Department staff members were skeptical. One of them asked, "Are you really as sick as they say you are?" My father implored them to call our trusted expert. The hospital staff answered that he is observing a holiday and is not available. My father did not relent. "It's our holiday, too. We need him." I don't know if Dr. Mankin really got a call. But the disposition of my case was to admit me to an inpatient bed for observation.

The medical school students and residents from multiple disciplines were very interested in my swollen abdomen. And when I heard them in the hallway discussing my case during morning rounds, I heard that I had some measure of celebrity because I was also a doctoral student.

Maybe it was because of the poking of my abdomen by so many people, or maybe it was because I watched the 1976 release of *Carrie* on television, or maybe it was because I had a fragile, distended spleen and low platelets, but I began to feel faint. And my abdomen felt vaguely uncomfortable, as if my condition could improve with a big belch.

On one trip to the toilet I felt lightheaded with a rushing sound in my ears. There was no one waiting outside and if I collapsed, there would be no immediate rescue. I took deep breaths, moved slowly, and opened the door. I don't recall how I got back to my room, but I surely had help from the nurses. My life experience had already taught me what a dangerous loss of blood feels like. I also appreciated the indispensability of good nurses.

The next day I had liver and spleen imaging. An internist came to my room to tell me that I was bleeding into my spleen, and the situation was becoming very serious. He told me that I needed surgery very, very soon to remove the spleen. A thoracic surgeon visited me. He told me that my platelet level was very low. He said that I would receive blood transfusions through the night to bring my platelets to a level safe enough for surgery. He added, "As soon as we clamp off the spleen your platelets will rise."

*

What I remember of the next day was waking up to surprises. I concluded that surgery always ends with surprises. My throat felt juicy and I wanted to cough. But I felt as though my abdomen was going to explode with the pain. A surgical resident who visited me said casually, "You're going to be lighter." And he indicated that it would be a while before I could eat because "We had to monkey with your digestive system." With a little more elaboration I understood that part of my intestines had been taken out of my body to allow access to the spleen, and were then reinstalled. And I understood that the removed spleen was quite large.

I recall having a visitor the next day. The nurses had me out of the bed, sitting on a soft chair. I held a pillow against my mid-section while I tried to cough. A thin man in a suit and a bowtie came in, and introduced himself as a Gaucher Disease researcher. He reported to me that the current state of Gaucher Disease research suggested that the field was on the verge of significantly helping people. He asked if I would be willing to allow him to take possession of my spleen, now elsewhere in the building. I thought, "I've already made this donation," but I simply said, "of course. You can have anything you want." He indicated that he would want some of my laboratory results and I was very happy to provide consent for that too.

The scientist sat in an available chair, crossed his legs, and began to talk about his Gaucher Disease research. He said that one of the ethical dilemmas that he faced was with the newly developed prenatal test. "Parents can abort their fetuses," he said, "but the problem is that all of the Gaucher people I meet are smart, productive people, like you. What do you think about this? What should I do?" I said that, as a researcher, he was only providing knowledge, and the ethical dilemma really belongs to the people contemplating termination of a pregnancy. The point was not lost on me, however, that he was stating that the broader implication of the tests that he was developing was that I myself might not have been born if the test had been available years earlier.

I held the pillow tighter against my mid-section and added, somewhat rudely, "I've wanted for a long time to meet someone like you, but not on the day after surgery." He understood immediately and invited me to visit his research laboratory when I was feeling better. Nevertheless, I was very pleased for my first opportunity to meet a Gaucher Disease researcher. And I noted that this person was pensive regarding both the good and bad implications of his work. He seemed to be smart as well as morally principled. I was glad to see that we had a person of this caliber working on the problems of Gaucher Disease. I wished that I would someday feel well enough to continue our discussion.

*

When my splenectomy's surgical dressing was changed, I got my first look at what had transpired to allow me to separate from my spleen. An incision started high on my chest and extended to a place low on my abdomen. Over the incision were big loops of black synthetic strands that seemed to be nylon. The surgical resident said that these were called retaining sutures. They were individually knotted and apparently acted like big clamps to hold me shut. These big loops were clear evidence that my wound was much more than skin-deep. Below the retaining sutures, the surface of the skin was sewn shut with thin strands of a black thread.

One evening, Dr. Mankin visited me. He said that he was there to wish me a good *Yom Kippur* and that he was on his way to synagogue because, he said, in a tone that was unmistakably wry, "I'm so religious." I held the pillow against my abdomen although it really did little for the pain. "You," he added, "do not have to fast. You have special dispensation." I was right with him on that point and replied, "I feel no need to afflict myself any further."

Soon after *Yom Kippur*, I was discharged to my parents and I stayed at their house in my familiar surroundings. I saw the skin growing around the knots of the retaining sutures. The wound was painful and I felt continuously miserable. Two weeks later my Dad and I drove to Boston for a post-surgical follow-up. As I was lying on the surgeon's examining table, he cut the skin sutures and picked out the small threads with a shiny instrument. Next he cut the retaining sutures just above the knots. He seemed to get a good grip on the retaining suture highest on my chest. I was staring at the ceiling tiles. He gave the nylon loop a hard pull. Then he grasped the next one and did the same. Then he pulled the next one, and the one after that, and the one after that. After pulling out half of them he stopped, looked me in the eye and asked, "How are you doing?" "Fine," I said calmly, which was completely true. He continued along the line of nylon loops, pulling them all out with firm, deliberate movements.

When he was done, I saw a pile of these thick strands on the tray next to me. There were a few drops of blood on my skin, which he covered with gauze pads. Without the retaining sutures, I felt immediately better than I had upon entering the office. And I confirmed something about neuroanatomy. My surgical incision was vertical, just to the left of the midline of my abdomen. My peripheral nerves were cut during the surgery, leaving the area between the incision and the midline quite numb. I seem to have achieved a pain-reducing side effect from the surgery. Removal of these sutures did not hurt, even though I felt inexplicably better after they were gone. My father was surprised to hear me suggest that we should go somewhere nice for lunch.

12.

Back at school, people welcomed me with genuine affection. But they were quietly appalled by how bad I looked. My major advisor, an important person in the life of a PhD student, told my best friend, Sheldon, to keep an eye on me. I was still recovering from infectious mononucleosis. It was a real diagnosis this time, not like the false positive during kindergarten. But I had also lost a lot of blood and had endured abdominal surgery.

Our learning disabilities professor was well known by all of the students to be a formidable scholar. Other professors in the department seemed to defer to her. Our major advisor told Sheldon and me to become very familiar with *phonemic segmentation*, the linguistic basis for the acquisition of reading and, therefore, also for developmental dyslexia. This was a specialty of our learning disabilities professor. The advice from our major advisor was that anything less than full knowledge of this concept prior to the learning disabilities course could potentially go badly. We were aware that any faculty member who thought that we were undeserving of the highest academic degree could appear at our dissertation defenses. The doctoral dissertation defense is where success or failure with achieving the degree is determined. Nobody needs a critical professor to show up, asking tough questions.

This respected but feared professor was also an extremely well regarded researcher. Her study demonstrating the underlying process for reading acquisition had been published in a highly regarded neuropsychology journal. She was the only member of the department's faculty whose work had been accepted into this peer-reviewed publication. Within the department, this journal was her territory.

My course in learning disabilities was scheduled for the early evening. During one such evening I sat in the front row as our professor droned on from the lecture notes she had used from that podium for the last thousand years. Early evening can be a difficult time to focus upon academic material, even without the added challenges of splenectomy, loss of blood, and infectious mononucleosis. The professor occasionally glanced up from her lecture notes and saw me in the front row, barely staying awake. I learned something important that evening about the power of suggestion.

"Let's stop early," she said, "I'm tired."

*

Weeks later Sheldon and I were preparing for her final exam. If I wrote a paper and did well on the exam, I could get an 'A' in the course. If I decided to take only the final exam, the best grade possible was a 'B.' Anything less than a 'B' is a failing grade in graduate school. I was very confident approaching the final exam. With everything else I had endured that semester I was eager to reduce my academic requirements. Do you know what they call a psychologist who got a 'B' in his learning disabilities course? They call him "doctor."

Sheldon and I worked together on our advisor's research, and some research of our own. With our advisor's encouragement, we worked to replicate a previously published neuropsychological study, with a few improvements to the research design. The plan was to submit our paper to the same neuropsychology journal that had earlier published the paper by our learning disabilities professor. "You won't get published there," our advisor cautioned us, "but at least we'll get a few good reviews of the paper that we can use to revise it, so that it can be published somewhere else."

*

Months later I visited the laboratory of the scientist I met the day after my splenectomy. This was a research center affiliated with an institution for persons with mental retardation. It was then that I began to appreciate the place held by Gaucher Disease among those disorders that affect the nervous system. My scientist-friend asked if I would be willing to provide a plug of skin from which he could clone the recently discovered mutation responsible for Gaucher Disease. I was nervous, but I had told him on the day after my splenectomy that he could have whatever he might want, and a promise is a promise.

During this visit I had the opportunity to see the scattergram plot of enzyme levels from many people. I was quite fluent by that time in the tools of science, including the methods of measurement and probability. I looked at the numbers related to the measured enzyme levels of his research sample, including the statistics relating to the variability of those numbers. I was shocked. The variability of this biochemical testing was far more extreme than the variability of psychological testing. No reputable psychological test of group membership would derive a result that could mean any of the possible conclusions. The statistical distributions of results from Gaucher non-carriers, Gaucher carriers, and individuals with Gaucher Disease overlapped considerably. Some test results could mean any of the possibilities.

*

I had recently taken a date to see the newly released *Superman* movie. There is a humorous scene in the movie where Superman's secret identity, Clark Kent, cannot open a soda bottle. Finally, with Lois Lane's help, the bottle opens and Clark spills soda and looks foolish. Lois looks at Clark and says, "Any more at home like you?" We, in the audience, know that Superman has no siblings and that his home planet, with his parents aboard, has blown up. Clark Kent, played by Christopher Reeve, adjusts his glasses and says, "Uh, n-no, not really." It's funny. Our doctoral advisor employed a research assistant named Kay, who was assigned to help us with our neuropsychological research project. She was smart, nice, and cute. But she was married. At an opportune moment I asked Kay, "Any more at home like you?" She said that she had a sister who was a graduate student in Philadelphia.

Kay found a way to introduce me to her sister Sue at a professional conference organized by my major advisor. Then Kay invited me to have dinner at her house that evening. Things seemed to go well between the sister and me, even if I did say at one point that my primary life focus at the moment was to finish graduate school. It's no wonder that doctoral students are socially isolated, with pronouncements like that one. But Sue stayed in touch anyway.

*

I was accustomed to hearing big news from Sheldon. He had recently announced that he was getting married. Then he announced that he had won a substantial prize in the state lottery. Then he announced that he was using his lottery winnings to purchase a half-interest in a racehorse, a trotter actually. Then he announced that his horse had been reduced in her classification and was entered in a race where she had a very good chance of winning.

Sheldon and I drove for hours to a small track in Pennsylvania. Our advisor gave Sheldon a few dollars to get in on the action.

The horse drew the number three post position, won by three lengths, and my $68 in gambling winnings represented a third of my monthly budget.

Some time later there was more big news from Sheldon that would enhance our status within the department. We were both on the line as we got our advisor on the phone.

"I have some really good news," Sheldon began.

"Did the horse come in again?" asked our professor.

"Better," I chimed in.

Sheldon was the one to speak. "Our paper was accepted."

Our professor was ecstatic. It was *his* graduate students who had pulled off this coup and had a paper published in the neuropsychology journal.

Sheldon and I sat together in the second semester of advanced statistics. This is where we learned how to use inferential statistics to predict the future. There are different kinds of relationships between variables. Sometimes, one variable changes in a very regular way as another variable changes, like the height of men and the length of their trousers. A graph of men's heights and the length of the trousers they buy (or the length of the trousers that their wives buy for them) would be a straight line. This linear relationship has certain mathematical properties that can be expressed by the formula that defines a straight line. More variables can be added to the equation to add to the precision of a prediction. We can even compute how likely we are to be right. And this is how that sinister $y=mx+b$ formula reappeared in my life, and then showed me one of the paths of science. It's one of the formulas for truth.

The point was not lost on Sheldon and me that the procedures of inferential statistics that we were studying with great success, the science of prediction, could be very lucrative at the track. Sheldon reviewed some of the research literature and discovered that we were not the first graduate students to think of this. Unfortunately, the variables involved in horse races are statistically unreliable. The numbers are too changeable, and there may be factors that are not published in the racing program. Horses can have bellyaches, drivers can be distracted — any number of things. I would recall this example years later when my goal was to quantify the variables predictive of success in a hospital treatment program. And, I would later learn, prediction of suicide is similarly statistically difficult, because human factors are so variable.

*

We received genuine praise from our learning disabilities professor following publication of our research study. She was demanding of her students because she wanted them to be at the top of their field. In that respect she reminded me of Dr. Mankin who, according to a newspaper article that I read during those years, delighted in seeing his students' abilities exceed his own. Great teachers can exist at any educational level, and in many different settings.

13.

A year later, our study became part of the literature review for the research that I would publish as my doctoral dissertation. I knew the methods of empirical inquiry. And I knew that a good scientist should be humble about his findings and be critical of his own work. I prepared to defend my results at an event advertised publicly within the university as *The Final Oral Examination of Wayne David Rosenfield, BA, MS, PDAS, Candidate for the Degree of Doctor of Philosophy.*

I had mastered the attributes of humility and self-criticism before I began to prepare for my dissertation defense. As I defended my research to an imaginary audience, I performed especially well in the role of people ripping my study to pieces. I was debating against myself, and I was losing. Three days before my dissertation defense, on a Saturday night, I was an emotional mess. I could see all of the weaknesses in my research design and all of the reasons why my dissertation defense on Tuesday would be a disaster.

Sue had, by now, finished her own degree and was living in Connecticut, with Kay and her husband, not far from campus. She had stuck around, despite my graduate student nerdiness. She was aware of my distress in preparing for my dissertation defense. Always practical, she said simply "You can't go on like this," and announced that we were going to the movies. We saw *Airplane!* which struck me as so funny that I could barely catch my breath. It was what I needed.

*

On Tuesday morning my publicly advertised dissertation defense was attended by my three doctoral advisors and by Sheldon. I stated the research problem, reviewed relevant past work published by researchers around the world, stated my research hypotheses, described my research design, and reported my results. Then I began to discuss the implications of my study for the research problem, and my recommendations for future studies. My major advisor began to ask me questions. I turned to the pile of books and journals to my left, which had many colored pieces of paper sticking out. For each possible question pertaining to the validity of my study I had prepared an answer, with a relevant reference. My advisor continued to fire questions at me. I was prepared. I had an answer for every question. I responded in a manner true to empirical principles.

My advisor picked up his copy of my dissertation and began to sign his name. I looked at my watch. The examination had lasted one hour and forty-five minutes. One of the other professors, the one I wasn't worried about, asked, "Don't we need to discuss?" My major advisor said, "Naaa," and handed his copy of my dissertation to the other two who, without any further questions, added their signatures to all of the necessary copies. I don't recall what else was said. But my professors had accepted my dissertation. Then they left. Sheldon and I packed up my books and papers.

My parents did not have any firsthand experience with the university world. But they knew that what was scheduled to happen today was a big part of my academic life. There is an old comedy bit popular in my family where a person says, "Call me a taxi," and the response is, "OK, you're a taxi." I called my parents' house from the payphone in the building. My Mom answered. "Call me a doctor," I said. My Mom seemed to be much more aware of the importance of the day than I realized, and she gushed with enthusiasm.

I thought of my grandfather, whom I had acknowledged in my dissertation. The surviving remnant of my family had escaped the Europe of the early twentieth century and, without money, or knowledge of English, or formal education, traveled to the other side of the world. They brought only themselves and their values. My grandfather did not see me become a *Bar Mitzvah*, but I knew that he would have been proud of me when I did. And then he would have been proud of me in a different way when I became a Doctor of Philosophy. Mostly, though, he simply expected me to be a *mensch*.

Sheldon and I walked to the Graduate School office with the signed copies of my dissertation. I found the clerk who needed to receive them. "Well," she asked animatedly, "are we a doctor?" I was emotionally spent, but smiled and simply said, "Yes."

*

Six months later Sheldon was my Best Man, and Kay was Sue's Maid of Honor, at a Colonial-era New England inn, under an evergreen *huppah*.

14.

I went to work as one of the psychologists for a school system in a moderately affluent town in Connecticut. For some of my time I was assigned to the middle school. I took this position the same year as a new administrator who was starting a second career. It was immediately apparent to both of us that we were very different people. He had just retired from a career as a military officer. He was regimented and organized. He seemed to expect the students and staff to be as organized as he was, and this caused friction between him and the faculty. He was usually, but not always, respectful in his dealings with me. He seemed to have little comprehension of the daily struggles of an adolescent with a disability. I thought that this was something with which I had some experience.

Most of the disabilities that we encountered in the public schools were invisible. Children with disabilities of an emotional, cognitive, or behavioral nature may evidence their problems in ways that look very much like misbehavior or contempt for authority. This type of response was not well received by the former military officer. My way of thinking often seemed to be closer to that of the adolescents in the building than to the administrator. I recalled my own revulsion at being told on my first day of college that I would be shining buttons.

My administrator friend seemed to be uncomfortable in this environment. He informed me, "I've just come from experiences that were very real." I had been through some experiences that were also "very real," and I saw parallels between my experiences and the challenges faced by some of the students. I stated, not very eloquently or convincingly at the time, that the daily life of the handicapped child was just as real to him, with a few important differences. The child didn't volunteer to be in this position. He had no prior training. When he was called upon by a superior to perform, he was all-alone, he could not call for help, there was no hope of rescue, and he could not resign from the requirements placed upon him. When he was successful, no one commended his bravery with a medal conferred in a formal ceremony. He wore no ribbons on his chest. The former officer and I saw things differently.

Although I had much experience as the recipient of professional services, I didn't speak about my own background. As a young professional, I knew my information. But in addition to being faithful to my profession and to my personal values, I wanted acceptance. I respected the advice that I was still relatively inexperienced, even if I did have an impressive degree.

The requirement for children with disabilities to get an educational program that was appropriate to their needs was now canonized in state and federal law. At planning meetings for children with all manner of disabilities, I was occasionally assertive. But I often deferred to the judgment of others. There were many people involved in these planning meetings, chaired by the former military officer. I was the only professional at the table with a doctorate. But the vast majority of these people were older than I was, more assertive than I was, and very often much more aggressive than I was. They had more years of experience than I did and they had strong opinions. I may have had an opinion about what a child needed, but I listened to other opinions politely and often went along with them.

There was a child who came to our attention who was a discipline problem, quite a thorn in the side of the administrator and many teachers. He was doing poorly academically and was often caught in class involved with behaviors of an antisocial nature. He wasn't doing anything really serious, nothing that would cause property damage or bodily harm to anyone. His behavior was prankish and he clowned in class in a manner that was annoying to the teachers. He disrupted the classroom environment, and the teachers demanded a solution.

There was uniform consensus that this young man was brighter than most of the other students in his classes. He showed comprehension of the subject matter. When he did the homework, it was of high quality. I knew that this adolescent had difficult circumstances at home. I thought that perhaps giving him a role of responsibility and leadership in an activity with his peers, led by a sensitive and caring adult, would give him the personal validation and social acknowledgement that he seemed to need. Maybe he could be engaged with coaching younger children, or maybe he could be engaged in an extracurricular activity or sport that would give him success and recognition. I spoke of these ideas to the members of the planning team. My ideas were received politely, but didn't catch fire.

Another idea was advanced during the planning meeting that if the young man were to be placed into more challenging classes, his time would be consumed by the increased demands of the homework and studying, and he would have less time for bad behavior. There was agreement that the student was intellectually capable of the more challenging classes. This idea seemed to appeal to the members of the planning team.

Several months later, the discussion at a follow-up meeting reported that the student's behavior had not improved. Even worse, he was now failing three classes. He felt more poorly about himself, and the school year was going badly for him. "Of course," I thought. "Why would anyone think that increasing academic demands is a solution for a child who feels poorly about his competency?" I recalled how I felt, years earlier, when I was over placed in my math classes. This plan, now shown to be seriously flawed, was a bad idea from the start. I looked at the signature page of the plan that had been implemented. I was shocked and appalled. There was my signature. I had approved this plan.

I felt awful. I thought, "I knew better than this. Why did I go along with a group decision that was so poorly conceived?" I concluded that I had signed-off on this plan for the most selfish of reasons: I wanted to be an accepted member of the group. I didn't want to be the one person in the room to say that the emperor has no clothes. "Never again," I thought. "They don't like me any better because I went along with them."

*

But I still cared too much about the opinions of others. On a couple of different inpatient treatment teams in the years that followed, I was present when our team psychiatrists behaved badly. One was insolent and disrespectful to a family member for no good reason that I was able to see. Another one publicly confronted and humiliated a nurse when he disagreed with her well-intentioned actions in dealing with a situation involving a patient. I didn't defend either of these people. And eventually I was the target of both of these overly self-important, highly credentialed professionals. "Never again," I thought one more time. Since then, I have chosen my battles carefully, evaluated situations with as much rationality as I can muster, and have responded with social propriety but unmistakable assertiveness. And I have been much more satisfied with my work, and with myself.

15.

Settling into our careers, my wife and I bought a house, and then another one. We had the space and financial security now to add children to our life. We thought that a prudent action would be to test my wife for the presence of the Gaucher mutation. Decoding of genes was not yet possible but there was a way to determine a person's Gaucher status. The scientist I had met the day after surgery could test blood for the presence of the key enzyme. The full expected amount of enzyme in a person's blood would indicate that the person has no mutated genes for the key substance. Half of the expected enzyme amount would indicate one mutated gene, or carrier status. And a low amount of enzyme would be expected in the blood of a person with Gaucher Disease.

My wife had her blood drawn at a hospital near our home in Connecticut. The sample was packed and shipped according to the instructions of the scientist. I considered this to be simply a formality. My wife joined the Jewish people prior to our wedding, and is not of Ashkenazi genetic descent. Nevertheless, within her European family's history was a name that could be Ashkenazi Jewish. There was some possibility that she had an Ashkenazi Jewish ancestor. Still being quite pleased about my survival of advanced statistics, knowing a few things about probability theory, and having seen the data from the testing procedure, I thought the chance of her having a Gaucher mutation was so low as to be barely worth discussing.

The results suggested that she was a carrier. My wife was scared. I was most definitely unimpressed with that result. Having seen the statistics for these tests, I thought that this conclusion deserved a great deal of skepticism. We drove to the laboratory and the researcher drew her blood right there, amidst the very equipment that he would use to test it. This time the result showed her enzyme level to be well into the unaffected range. Science is good for a lot of things, including telling us when we shouldn't worry.

*

We were no longer anxious about having a child with Gaucher Disease. But being able to have a child at all was a growing concern. We had a diagnosis of *unexplained infertility*. We had a house, two careers, sufficient financial resources to support children, and we had each other. A child was deeply wanted, and would be guaranteed a good home. The irony, we quipped, is that to have the resources to comfortably support a family, we were now past the ages of greatest fertility. Other couples our age were having similar problems. Infertility is frustrating and, for people who want children in their lives, thoroughly heartbreaking.

Now, with *unexplained infertility*, I informed my urologist that I had been told about a varicocele prior to my summer on *Kibbutz Kinneret*. He said that a varicocele is a very common occurrence among men and results in a higher temperature where the sperm are made. Like Atlantic salmon who originate in their Canadian ancestral homelands, the most athletic swimmers are born in a slightly cooler environment. The urologist described the surgery that would correct this. I was no stranger to surgery and this seemed like a minor procedure.

"There is no *minor surgery*," said my urologist, "just *minor surgeons*. A good surgeon has to be ready for anything." I was glad to hear that he took his job so seriously. This was to be a small abdominal incision, near my waist. I didn't see this as a big deal. I had much experience already with surgeries that really were very big deals. I had no qualms.

I had the surgery. True to my expectation, I never needed any pain medicine. To me, this was minor surgery. I discussed it freely among my friends, at least one of whom needed the same procedure. "No big deal," I told him. Several weeks later I met my friend at the dry cleaners. "Wayne, you son of a bitch, how could you say that this surgery didn't hurt? I've never been in so much pain in all my life!"

I have no explanation for his bad experience. We did have the same surgeon. But everyone's body is different. Perhaps my *pain meter* has become re-calibrated. Did I really feel less pain than my friend? Or do we think and react differently to a similar pain stimulus? I have no answer for this. After many years as a psychologist, I am still amazed by the extent of differences between people.

*

Still, Sue and I had no pregnancy. We saw more doctors, and contemplated the procedures that would involve the female apparatus. These would be more invasive and painful, and some would not be covered by insurance. The expense would be akin to paying for another degree, but with far less chance of success. Then, unexpectedly, Sue had a positive pregnancy test.

I began a new job in a residential facility for persons with mental retardation who had concurrent behavioral and psychiatric problems. I had not been at work for very long one day, when I received a telephone call from my sister-in-law, Kay. She and Sue were at the hospital. My wife needed immediate surgery.

I didn't fall down the stairs rushing to leave the facility, but it was close. I drove quickly to the hospital, but missed seeing Sue prior to surgery. Apparently, the pregnancy had been ectopic, growing in the wrong place. It was acutely painful to her and was now creating a dangerous situation. The pregnancy needed to come out.

Kay was with me in the hospital room, when my unconscious wife, her sister, the one at home just like her, was wheeled back from surgery. We hugged and cried.

I felt profoundly lonely. Sure, I had my wife and her sister in the room with me. But in the earlier hours of that day, our lives were different. This early pregnancy would have been just a small group of cells, with little to differentiate it as human, and without a heartbeat. But it was so deeply wanted, that I felt that I had lost a person.

Our hopes of having children in the house seemed even more distant. We continued to consult doctors. We even visited the Tomb of Rachel. Both approaches are reportedly associated with fertility.

*

Just over a year later, I reported to Dr. Mankin that the hip he had repaired during the summer between high school and college was becoming quite painful. My walking range was limited. He had earlier advised me to wait as long as possible before considering a hip replacement, and I was fine with that. I was most definitely not a fan of undergoing surgery. But the degeneration of the hip that was repaired fifteen years earlier was starting to interfere with everyday activities. We agreed on a date in early March for replacement of my hip.

I've had an affinity with the space program since those early days of watching television with my mother when I was at home instead of attending kindergarten. Exposure to a conspicuously inspiring and technical adventure such as space exploration created my early excitement with science. The mission to send an American citizen into orbit aboard the space shuttle *Challenger* caught my attention. And the astronaut's role as the first public school teacher to give a lesson from space had the potential to inspire a new generation of students to pursue advanced education. The teacher was a fellow New Englander, from a New Hampshire town north of Boston. There was a low probability of a catastrophic failure of this flight. But the probability of a disaster was greater than zero. Man plans and God laughs. The destruction of the spacecraft and the loss of the entire crew was a national tragedy.

Four weeks after the loss of the *Challenger*, Sue again had a positive pregnancy test. We needed to be certain that this pregnancy was normal before proceeding with my hip replacement. A sonogram would be necessary to confirm that all was well. As the radiologist pronounced, "There's Junior," the sonogram revealed a blob on the screen, pulsating inside its uterine home.

Two weeks later Sue brought me to Boston for my planned hip replacement surgery. My parents met us there. They had been through the prior surgery experiences with me, and they were quite vigilant for my safety. My wife had a great deal of morning sickness, and was carrying their precious first grandchild. My parents hovered over her relentlessly and obsessively worried about me. I, of course, was the only player in this drama who had the benefit of anesthesia.

I awoke from surgery feeling better than I had earlier in the day. I had no anesthesia side effects, and there was no pain coming from my hip. I had come to expect awful surprises from surgery, but on this occasion I had a pleasant surprise. I alternated between sleep and wakefulness that evening. During a period of consciousness I caught part of a Boston television program entitled "Remembering Christa," about the teacher from New England who was lost aboard the *Challenger*.

The day after surgery, I greeted Dr. Mankin at my bedside, as he performed morning rounds with perhaps a half dozen medical students. I was still feeling fine. I was aware of the presence of the students, but my interaction was only with my doctor. I had the impression that the students were intimidated by him. None of them spoke. None of them asked questions. Their faces were solemn. They revealed no outward emotion or animation. In contrast, the Gaucher Expert was loud, animated, and clearly assertive and in control.

I was also aware of a lot of blonde and straight hair in the crowd. Dr. Mankin's black Ashkenazi mustache distinguished him from them even more than the differences in age and demeanor. The newspaper article that I had read several years earlier while I was at the University of Connecticut, mentioned that it was no longer unusual to see a Jewish doctor in the Boston academic community, seated as a full professor.

On this first morning after surgery, Dr. Mankin tried to get a good measure of my leg lengths. He stretched a tape measure from my right iliac crest to my right ankle. Then he measured the left leg the same way. The measurements kept showing that my right leg, the side that had the new hip, was longer than the left leg. He said, "That can't be right, they were the same in the operating room." Dr. Mankin was happy to write this off as a measurement error here in my hospital bed and of no real significance. But he turned to the students, and said in his best Barbra Streisand voice, "Sam, you made the leg too long." Not missing my cue, I pointed my thumbs to my upper chest and said, "The lapels are fine, though." We both howled with laughter. The students were silent, looking very uncomfortable.

The next day we repeated the same *shtick*. We both laughed. Students were silent. The leg lengths were perfect, as expected.

16.

I went home with my wife. I observed the prescribed new-right-hip maintenance conditions of no flexion beyond ninety degrees, no internal rotation, and no adduction past the midline. In everyday language this means lying on the left side with a pillow between my knees. Dr. Mankin advised me to avoid jarring the hip, for now and into the future. If I take care of it, I was told, the hip should last for many years.

I watched hours upon hours of television during this early post-surgical time, and about two minutes of that time is noteworthy as an influence upon my career.

I watched the hearings of the Rogers Commission, a public investigation into what had happened to the *Challenger*. I enjoyed the demonstration by physicist Richard Feynman, PhD, who used a small piece of rubber, his ice water, and two fingers to reproduce the mechanical problem that destroyed our spaceship. He demonstrated that scientific truth can be confirmed and the results can be reproduced, a key part of the philosophy that underlies empirical inquiry.

I also watched dozens of movies. Sue brought home a steady supply of VHS cartridges which enabled me to occupy many hours meaninglessly. One movie which had an intelligent premise and was very well acted was titled "...and justice for all," starring Al Pacino. I won't spoil the movie's ending for anyone about to have hip replacement surgery, but near the end of an extended climactic scene, the main character, an early career lawyer, is heard yelling to an older professional with poor ethical standards, "You're supposed to stand for something!" I liked that. I thought about what it means to adhere to the standards of a profession. I concluded that, although a person is mortal, fallible, and imperfect, at the moment that he is in a professional role, he has a responsibility to that role. A psychologist, for example, is expected to act at all times for the benefit of the client or patient. There cannot be any dual allegiance or any motive other than to do what is in the client's or patient's best interest. Any less than full adherence to this standard is destructive to the profession.

*

Our son, Aaron, was born about six weeks early. My mother in law remarked, "That's the smallest baby I've ever seen," as he fit into the crook of my elbow. He seemed so fragile, and I felt very protective. During at least one night I fell asleep listening to his breathing on the baby monitor. Because he was so small, he needed to be fed every two hours. By alternating responsibility, Sue and I could each get four consecutive hours of sleep. We wondered if younger parents have more stamina for infant care. We were exhausted.

Aaron was bundled tightly for trips outside during the New England winter, and for a flight to Chicago. His maternal great grandfather, born before there were airplanes, laughed uproariously when I told him that Aaron already had a frequent flier account.

During the spring Sue had some familiar symptoms. She sent me out in the evening to buy a pregnancy test. We stood over Aaron's crib and watched him as he slept. This infant who did not even dent the mattress would be a big brother.

David was born into the New England winter. The workload for taking care of two babies is enormous. Maybe it would have been nice to be younger for this task. I didn't see how it would even be possible without the new hip.

In the residential treatment facility where I worked, there were many strongly religious staff persons. I'm flattered when people tell me that they have prayed for me in their own religion. I accept the gesture as an expression of human concern. One of the staff persons revealed to me that, during the time that my wife and I seemed to be unable to have a child, "I was praying for you." "You can stop now," I answered. "It's getting to be kind of a problem."

*

Three years later, as my wife and I prepared to bring our two toddlers to a shopping mall for the first time, I told my older son, "If you get lost, find a policeman." I remembered the scene from that significant movie during my springtime on the couch. And I thought, "I hope the policeman is all right." I was relying upon the integrity of an unknown professional for the safety of my children. If we cannot confidently rely upon that integrity, we are sunk as a society.

17.

I then had a period of five years that was my Golden Age of Gaucher. I had a pain-free hip. I walked well. I had occasional nosebleeds, but my Gaucher Disease was not a problem. I could focus upon my work and upon my very busy household. I could ignore Gaucher Disease once again.

My father and I attended a meeting of the National Gaucher Foundation, in Bethesda, Maryland. I think this was the first meeting of its kind, with affected people and their families, professionals, and the executive staff persons from a tiny new company that was developing a treatment.

The meeting was also attended by perhaps two dozen people with Gaucher Disease, more or less. Some of the women wore maternity clothing, not because they were pregnant, but because they wanted to cover their spleen filled abdomens. Two young parents sat in front of my father and me. The mother was astonished to hear me introducing myself as a person with Gaucher Disease. They were attending the meeting, she informed us, because they were told that their toddler at home with Gaucher Disease would die soon. They were there, courageously, to learn as much as possible. The potential of a different outcome was not previously known to them.

We met the mother of a young child named Abby, who lived in Massachusetts not far from my parents. Abby was at home, suffering with recurrent and excruciating bone pain. Abby's mother, too, had been told of a limited life expectancy for her child. Other participants walked painfully with assistive devices, or were carried.

The president of the NGF began his remarks to those assembled. "It works. It works. It works," he said. He was referring to the enzyme replacement therapy currently in development, still two years from commercial availability. There was a palpable atmosphere of optimism in the room.

We all joined together for a cocktail party and dinner in the evening. Not surprisingly, most people had a story of Gaucher Disease problems to relate. What I did find surprising was that the others and I were truly interested in everyone else's stories. Making connections with people who had experienced similar problems felt comforting, even empowering.

After the conference, in the terminal building at National Airport in Washington, my father and I again encountered the corporate people we had met. I watched the plane that was carrying essentially the entire company leave the ground. And I'm pretty certain that I whispered a prayer.

*

I continued to see Dr. Mankin every year. He was pleased with the stability of my hip. On the x-ray films he showed me where my bone was growing into the metal parts. He told me that the newly available medicine for Gaucher Disease seemed to be a good treatment. I tried to learn as much as I could.

I was nervous about being one of the first people to receive a new product on the cutting-edge of biotechnology. I consulted a hematologist. I asked about the report of recipients forming antibodies and what this could possibly mean for the course of my disease. I asked about hypothetical problems. The answer

I got was that there was insufficient knowledge at that time to give a definitive answer.

In graduate school, the process of reducing research problems to testable hypotheses taught me to respect science, but also to recognize the constraints upon what we can verifiably know. I learned that the most important questions are those that we don't know enough to ask. We often don't know what we don't know.

I asked the sales representative about the drug's safety, knowing that it was a product extracted from human tissue. He assured me that there were several purification steps in the drug's manufacture. He said, "There is no way" that an unknown disease could be transmitted by the medicine.

I thought about Donny, my roommate with hemophilia from three decades earlier. And I recalled a man whom I met in recent years who was a physician, husband and father. He received the new medicine for hemophilia years earlier, before *human immunodeficiency virus* had been discovered. The medicine was sold as an answer to a genetic disorder. But scientists didn't know what they didn't know. As a result, this man's life expectancy would be very short. I was glad that there was a treatment for Gaucher Disease. But I saw no reason to be one of the first people to try it.

The episodes of bone pain well known to people with Gaucher Disease were now identified medically as *bone crises*. These painful episodes occur when bone tissue is being strangled by the abundance of a fatty substance that accumulates in people with Gaucher Disease. This was the situation with Abby, the young daughter of the mother that my Dad and I met at the NGF meeting. Abby was extremely fatigued, had a very swollen abdomen, was experiencing abnormal bleeding, and endured episodes of unremitting bone pain. Abby was in the same hospital where I had a similar experience at roughly that age. I knew what she was going through. Her situation resonated with my family and me.

My father was a Freemason. He had been the Master of his Masonic lodge at least twice, and he was now in the Shriners. He found expression of his humane values in these groups. And the orthopaedic mission of the Shriners was meaningful to him for obvious reasons. When he came home one evening from a meeting, he asked his wife and children which unit of the Shriners he should join. There was no question in our minds that he should join the clowns. On one occasion, my Dad arranged to have a carload of clowns visit the home of a sick child.

My Dad was present for Abby's first infusion of the new medicine for Gaucher Disease. Having attended the meeting with my father and me two years earlier, Abby's mother kept watch on the drug approval process and pressed to get her daughter treated as soon as possible. Abby's mother was the lioness watching over her. After FDA approval, Abby's infusion was the first such administration of this medicine in New England. A representative from the pharmaceutical company was there, as well as a news crew from a local television station, and my Dad, who provided an interview for the evening news. I never knew my Dad to hide his emotions, and he cried as the new medicine dripped into Abby's intravenous line. Abby and her family had high hopes that she would finally get relief from these recurrent, unremitting, devastatingly painful bone crises. And of course, success for Abby would mean success for a lot of us. Maybe Abby would become a normal teenager and have a chance for a normal life.

*

Seventeen months after the drug was approved, I was not hearing any bad things about the new medicine. And I did hope to avoid any future Gaucher Disease related problems. I was ready to try it. But, as the saying goes, *"Mensch tracht und Gott lacht."* Man plans, and God laughs.

Abby was now almost a teenager, and she still endured significant Gaucher Disease symptoms. Despite having more energy, she had bone crises that seemed to be increasing in frequency. She too was subjected to suggestions by her physicians that she was complaining needlessly or was crying "for attention."

Planning was underway for a meeting of the National Gaucher Foundation, in Newark, New Jersey. There would be a part of the meeting just for children and I was asked to lead it. I was looking forward to another opportunity to connect with the Gaucher community, especially now that the group had some experience with enzyme replacement therapy. Trying to maintain a semblance of normalcy, Abby planned to be present with me in Newark for the children's program. We would provide support together to children affected by Gaucher Disease.

I had been bicycling several times each week, for usual rides of five to fifteen miles, but sometimes longer. I was eating right, taking vitamins, and getting regular exercise. I entered the *Five Boro Bike Tour*, a ride of thirty-six miles on a Sunday morning through the streets of New York, originating in lower Manhattan near the twin towers of the World Trade Center.

I completed the *Vernon to Vernon Century*, a bicycle event of one hundred miles in a single day, from Vernon, Vermont to Vernon, Connecticut. My wife and sons met me at the finish where, with a loud "Oy!" I peeled myself off the seat. I felt that I was in the best physical condition of my life. Man plans and God laughs.

18.

I had noticed a bump on my left shin for several months, starting in the spring. It was out of place on my leg, like a hard blister under the skin. By summer, I noticed that the bump was starting to feel tender. I had an annual orthopaedic appointment scheduled for the early autumn, for regular observation of my metal right hip. I noticed that the bump was becoming increasingly uncomfortable, and that I was taking increasing amounts of pain medicine. I decided to advance my appointment by a few weeks so Dr. Mankin could look at it.

The appointment followed the usual pattern. On the orthopaedic clinic day, I visited the radiology department first, and brought the films to the office. My hip was fine. Then Dr. Mankin looked at the bump. The x-ray of my left shin showed an area of bone loss under the bump. To me it looked as though a bite had been taken out of the bone. Dr. Mankin drew fluid out of the leg for analysis. His experience with Gaucher bone taught him that the normal process of bone remodeling can be disrupted in Gaucher Disease. There was no obvious indication that this bump was anything more serious than that. But the bone would need to be repaired to prevent a fracture.

*

The surgery to repair the area of bone loss was scheduled for the following week. My most recent prior surgery, the hip replacement, was not a terrible experience. I had an optimistic view of the coming bone repair as the last Gaucher complication I would ever see prior to beginning enzyme replacement therapy.

In the preoperative area a physician identified himself as an anesthesiologist. We discussed the procedure that I was about to undergo, and I was relaxed. Once again I was aware of watching ceiling tiles as I was wheeled to a tiled hallway and parked outside of an operating room. A masked female came to my side and engaged me in a discussion related to the anesthesia that I would be receiving. "Are you a nurse?" I asked. She said, "No. I'm an anesthesiologist." I was confused. "I just met a guy who said that he was my anesthesiologist." The answer was sufficiently straightforward. "I'm his professor," said the masked woman.

We continued to chat. We discovered that we had a lot in common, including having been doctoral students at the University of Connecticut at about the same time, although on different campuses. A man greeted me, presumably an orthopaedic resident or fellow who was walking toward the entrance to the operating room. He said, "We'll see if it's what we think it is." "What a curious thing to say," I thought, "I'm here for a bone repair and then I'll be on my way." *Mensch tracht und Gott lacht.*

The anesthesiologist appeared over me again, this time unmasked, in the recovery room to say goodbye. I needed to be reminded who she was, perhaps because I was still disoriented from anesthesia. But I hadn't seen her face before, either.

*

I learned that evening that my tibia had not been repaired. My leg was in a cast. A biopsy had been taken. "Well," I thought, "that's certainly disappointing." I didn't understand why the situation was now different.

19.

Dr. Mankin told me that the reason for the bone loss was not entirely clear. He said it could be abnormal remodeling of Gaucher bone. Or, he said, it could be a malignancy. We would need to wait for the pathology report. Several days passed.

One evening Dr. Mankin appeared without warning, accompanied by one or two associates. I recall my parents being with me at the time. The pathology results were in, he said. "It's a sarcoma, a soft tissue cancer," he said. "You will need surgery, and some combination of radiation and chemotherapy. We don't know yet if you will have just radiation or just chemotherapy, or both. But you need more surgery for sure." And then the orthopaedists left.

The rest of the evening is a blur to me. An emotional bomb had just gone off. I was shocked. I remember feeling enormously scared. I felt numb. I felt that my world had just crumbled to pieces. Everything seemed to be unreal. I was overwhelmed. I recall no thoughts other than "I'm not done." I was frozen, not physically, but singularly focused upon what I had just been told. I didn't know what else to do. I recall few other details of the evening. I don't know if I received any medicine and I have no memory of my nighttime routine, when my parents left, who else I might have spoken to, how I got into bed, or whether I slept.

The next day, or some time during the next week — I really don't know — I had multiple scans and x-rays. I think I had some comprehension at the time that there was a search for metastases. My lungs would be a prime target for the spread of a sarcoma. I was emotionally numb. My thoughts turned to my sons, who were now ages six and four. And I thought that if I were to die now, I would become, in their lives, only an abstraction. They were so young. They would not know me as adults. They would not remember me.

When my wife and sons visited me in the hospital, the boys were curious about everything they saw. They were interested in the PCA pump, the device for patient controlled administration of morphine into my intravenous line. They took turns pushing the button. One of them asked, "Feel better, Dad?" They were becoming the humane, caring people I hoped they would. My heart ached at the thought that this would be what they would remember of me, and that this memory too would fade.

At some point Dr. Mankin was at my bedside. He, by then, knew the results of my many scans. "You have one lesion in your body," he said. "And," he added while pointing to my leg, "it's right there." I was comforted to hear this man, in whom I had unquestioning trust, say that the dimensions of the issue were now defined. I learned that I had an *angiosarcoma*.

*

One evening, a petite, very animated young woman appeared in my room. She introduced herself as an activity therapist. She said that there would be a barbecue "in the penthouse," and that I was invited. I pointed out to her that I had a cast on my leg, and that I was not cleared to walk on it. "That's ok," she said. "We'll send someone with a wheelchair to get you." I thought, "Well, I'm not doing anything else this evening," and I agreed to go. "What's the penthouse?" I asked. She answered that it is an activity area on a top floor of the hospital.

As promised, an older man wearing a smock arrived at the planned time in the evening to bring me to the barbecue. Our route was through many previously unseen hallways and an elevator that was also unfamiliar to me. He wheeled me into "The Penthouse," a large room crowded with many patients in wheelchairs. There was a large window and a door to an area outside, high above the city. The barbecue grill was in the outside area and the activity therapist was there, roasting chicken.

Navigation of this room was difficult, crowded with patients in wheelchairs, some with family members seated near them. I met a woman who seemed to be about my age who said that she too had an *angiosarcoma* and that she was also a patient of my doctor. She told me that her tumor was on her pelvis. I thought that the abdomen would be a bad place for a cancer. I thought that my own worst-case scenario would be to get rid of my sick leg if necessary. But a tumor on a pelvis was a different situation. She added that she had been in the hospital for months and hoped to be home before Christmas. "Well," I thought to myself, "that's not a good sign."

I met some people recovering from severe burns, including one man who had no nose or movement in his face, who moved about only by manipulation of a joystick on his electric wheelchair. Another man, his arms and hands immobilized and outstretched, said that he had been working around a fryer. Somehow his hands and arms had gotten immersed in the frying oil up to his elbows. I didn't press for details.

I was still feeling very emotionally damaged and vulnerable. But I smiled to myself about the irony of burn survivors attending a barbecue. Everyone seemed to be having a good time.

*

During the week I spoke by telephone with Abby. I told her that I certainly would not be attending the meeting in Newark. She seemed to be doing well, was currently free of bone pain, and would attend the meeting as planned. I said to her, "I don't know how or when, but I'm going to dance with you." She agreed.

20.

After my case was fully evaluated by multiple disciplines, I was discharged home with my wife. The treatment plan called for ten daily radiation treatments over two weeks, to be followed by surgery. Chemotherapy was not a meaningful treatment for survival of *angiosarcoma*, I was told, and was not recommended.

I drove myself to the Radiation Therapy Department every day, to a device called a linear accelerator. Walking with crutches was a familiar experience for me. Just like riding a bicycle, you don't forget.

Radiation therapy started as a simple experience. The technicians would position me on the table and leave the room. A small red light would come on for one minute and fifty-seven seconds. The light would go off, and the technicians would return to help me get up. Then I would leave and come back the next day to repeat the process. There was no sensation associated with the procedure.

After the fourth such treatment I felt exhausted. The level of fatigue reminded me of the infectious mononucleosis years earlier. I would arrive at the hospital early so I could nap in the car before going inside.

After several sessions I asked one of the technicians what type of radiation I was receiving. He said, "This is X-ray radiation, photon energy." I looked at the machine aimed at my leg. As the technicians were returning to the safety of the control room, leaving me to be alone with the beam of high intensity radiation, I said, "Standby to fire photon torpedoes!" The last technician to leave the room looked over his shoulder to see his weird patient. And suddenly I felt old.

These linear accelerator drivers were, I estimated, in their early twenties. They would have been born during or just after the years when I was watching *Star Trek* on television. I was just being me, weird humor and all. I hadn't read a book telling me how to survive cancer. I didn't know of any book that would have advised me. And I didn't yet know what a favor I was doing for myself by creating a mental image of my tumor as a Klingon battle cruiser about to be blasted by the photon torpedoes at our disposal.

But there was more. I sometimes thought of the tumor as the *Wicked Witch of the West*, and these high-energy photons represented the water that would destroy her.

This was war. The dimensions of the battle that was shaping up between this cancer and me were growing. I knew by now that I would be receiving a piece of donor bone. I learned that the bone I would receive was already identified in the bone bank. I gave blood over a period of two weeks, for storage, to be returned to my body during surgery if I needed it. And I was certain to eat enough blood-building food to restore the blood still in my body back to its full fighting strength. I didn't see any acceptable outcome other than victory. I was getting mad. And I thought, "My middle name is David! Bring on the uncircumcised Philistine!"

*

I contacted my orthopaedic anesthesiologist, whom I considered to be a part of my support team. We talked by telephone. I told her that my procedure was scheduled for the middle of November, and that I hoped she would be my anesthesiologist again. She listened to me and said simply, "Just do whatever Dr. Mankin says to do and you'll be ok." And she promised that, as my anesthesiologist, "I won't let anything bad happen to you." I believed her.

21.

Surgery was scheduled for the Monday before Thanksgiving. My wife and I stayed in a hotel near the hospital. We were at the surgery reception area before sunrise. Lying in the pre-operative area I met the anesthesiologist, who smiled and said that she was glad that she was on time.

The anesthesiologist said that she would be adding "a short acting benzodiazepine" to my intravenous line. I saw that there was also a large syringe attached to my line that presumably held something more potent. Before she could add the medicine, a woman arrived at my side and said that I hadn't yet signed consent for the procedure. The anesthesiologist took a step back and the woman spoke. She told me that I was about to have a procedure she named as "an allograft with muscle flap." I understood that I would have a tumor cut out, that my tibia would be replaced with a piece of donor bone, that the muscle from the back of my shin would be cut and flapped over the top to be reattached in a new position, and that skin would be taken from my thigh to graft over the wound. She stated aloud all of the bad things that could happen. I didn't believe a word of the bad stuff. I thought, "This is the last day that I will have any cancer in my body." She put a pen into my hand and my signature represented my informed consent.

The anesthesiologist stepped forward and added medicine to my line. I felt the relaxation spread throughout my body. After some period of time I told her that I would like more of that short acting benzodiazepine. She was happy to indulge my request.

I cannot accurately say how much time passed, but at some point the anesthesiologist grasped the syringe attached to my intravenous line, and my memory of that day ended.

*

My next awareness was of a window, and I saw that there was darkness outside. I cannot say for certain where I was at that time. At some point I was in a hospital bed. To my right was a window through which I could see the Boston skyline. I took note of the blue light at the top of the older John Hancock Building. Turning my head to the left I could see down a corridor that seemed to have busy nurses walking in various directions.

I was at a location notable for the extreme level of responsiveness of the entire nursing staff. I immediately observed that when I turned on my nurse call light, someone appeared right away, even a nurse who was not assigned to me. One nurse remarked to me during my time there that this ward dispenses "the most narcotics of any unit in the hospital, because bone surgery is the most painful." I suggest that another reason for the high rate of administration of opiate medicine on the unit is that this nursing staff was among the most compassionate. If they didn't respond to patients so diligently, they wouldn't be treating so much pain.

I was having an easy time. My pain level was quite manageable. I had no complaints. I was pleased with my good fortune, that I could have an extremely complex surgical procedure and still be so comfortable. I now considered myself to be an orthopaedic surgery patient, and not a cancer patient. Opening my eyes before sunrise, I spied Dr. Mankin at the end of the hall, already at work. I looked to my right and saw a flashing blue light on the John Hancock Building.

Dr. Mankin appeared at my bedside for morning rounds a few hours later with orthopaedic residents and fellows. Everyone seemed to be upbeat. My surgical team was pleased with the outcome of the procedure.

I was wheeled to the x-ray department for a look at my reconstructed leg. Before leaving, I asked if I could see the films. The donor bone looked like concrete next to my comparatively thin bone. There were many metal parts at both ends of the new bone. I imagined that the donor of this tissue must have been healthy and comparatively young, having died traumatically from a wound that left his lower body intact. My Dad said that he prayed for the comfort of my donor's family. On Wednesday I may have had more discomfort but I don't recall a terrible experience.

22.

The next day, Thursday, Thanksgiving Day, 1992, is burned into my memory as a day of unspeakable pain. My wound screamed at me from within. The sound of a voice in the room seemed to reverberate through my body, settling at the wound. Any movement, any sound, even the effort to form a thought, stimulated a bolt of stabbing pain from the wound. There was no comfortable position. The pain was searing and without respite.

I didn't know how I could survive this. My nurses called the Pain Service, a part of the Anesthesiology Department. A doctor appeared, whom I remember as Asian, with an animated, round face, and a broad smile. He seemed to like his work and I was pleased to see him. He offered an oral medicine and said that he would return in an hour.

This was the recurring pattern. Each hour seemed to be of endless duration. But the doctor from the Pain Service returned each time, as promised. I did not have any relief. At each hourly visit he offered ever more aggressive treatment. I cannot say for how many consecutive hours we continued this routine. To me it was agony without end. He consistently showed optimism and a cheerful demeanor. Finally, I received an injection of something, I don't know what, and I could rest, being careful not to move.

I never learned his name and I never saw him again. What I have, is a memory of him saying, in very heavily accented

English, "Ahh, Mister Rosenfeerd, you be home for Hanukah." I was amused. But I dared not to laugh. I thought then, and I have thought many times since, that if there are angels on Earth, they include this doctor and these nurses.

My parents were with me for part of the day. Sue arrived with our sons, who wanted to perform a puppet show for me. I wasn't a very good audience and they remarked that I was grouchy. The hospital provided a Thanksgiving meal, and there were two more meals brought by my family. I couldn't eat. I questioned what I could be thankful for on this traditional American holiday. I couldn't think of any blessings other than the people who were there with me. I thought that my life's blessings were totaled on one hand. By nighttime I had some relief. I could again foresee a life beyond the hospital bed.

23.

The nurses told me that the weather was turning cold. I looked out on the buildings of downtown Boston. The light on the John Hancock Building was red. I was sure it had been blue days earlier. When my night nurse came in to check on me, I asked her what medications they were giving me that could be altering my perception. She was puzzled by my question. She told me that I was not getting anything that was mind-altering. "Look at the light on the John Hancock Building," I implored. "What color is it?" She agreed that it was red, but had not noticed a blue light earlier in the week. I was certain that my perception was being affected chemically. I could think of no other explanation.

Later that night I opened my eyes. The light on the John Hancock Building was flashing red. When my nurse came in, we agreed that it was flashing red. If my perception was altered, then my nurse's perception was too. This mystery was an amusing diversion from how broken I was feeling.

*

In the coming days, my pain abated. "You've turned the corner," Dr. Mankin told me. Together we looked at my wound. I had known surgical wounds to be incisions, simple cuts that could be sewn together, like the splenectomy scar extending from my chest to my abdomen. This wound looked very dramatic. It was an oblong circular crater, bloody in places but otherwise black. There was a fine mesh appearance to its surface. On my thigh was a bloody mess that felt like the road-burn that I once experienced when I fell off my bicycle. One of the orthopaedic fellows explained to me that they had sliced the surface skin from that site to plant on top of the wound left by removal of the tumor, covering all of the other reconstruction. This skin donor site was not a deep wound. But it bled, which the surgeons insisted was a good sign.

Pulling my toes back caused the relocated muscle to flex noticeably inside my very impressive surgical wound. Clearly, my leg was never going to look the same as it had before, but that was acceptable to me. My situation seemed to be improving.

*

I was visited by a physical therapist who described the extensive rehabilitation that was ahead. Walking on this leg was going to take about a year. This felt like an ambush. I was shocked. This was not part of my plan. I told my nurse that I wanted to talk to my doctor. One of the orthopaedic residents arrived. I told her what the physical therapist had told me. The response of this orthopaedic resident was notable for its icy dearth of compassion. She took a sheet of paper from her clipboard, turned it toward me and said, "These are all the people I have to take care of." I felt my throat tighten and I thought I would cry. "They're all important," I squeaked. I don't know if I thanked her for coming, but I was surely glad to see her leave.

I told my wife what had happened with the orthopaedic resident. There were some events of which I have no firsthand knowledge. But when I told Sue that this particular resident was no longer in the group that made rounds in the morning, she replied "Oh, really?" The lioness had pounced.

*

I told my sister about my observations of the light on the older John Hancock Building. She did a little research and found some interesting information. She told me that the architect of the building wanted to create a beacon, perhaps like the navigation beacon that once existed on the high ground of Boston for the benefit of mariners. Beacon Hill is now quite the high rent district. This current beacon, visible from much of Boston, is maintained by a local radio station. This poem is less well known than the one about Paul Revere, and I don't think that Massachusetts pupils are required to learn it:

Steady blue, clear view.
Flashing blue, clouds due.
Steady red, rain ahead.
Flashing red, snow instead, or, during summer, the Red Sox game is rained out at Fenway.

That doesn't completely rhyme. Not everything in Massachusetts makes sense.

24.

During the second week after surgery I was fitted with a brace to immobilize my leg and I went home with Sue. We felt overwhelmed with the task of caring for this wound. And Sue was also caring for two young children while working full time.

Three weeks later the wound was increasingly painful. And it seemed to be more moist than I remembered. There was enough brown liquid to fill the wound crater and even to spill out. I called the orthopaedic service. The advice was to return to Boston immediately.

The orthopaedic fellow who looked at the wound said that it was infected. The plan would be to admit me to the hospital and to clean the wound surgically the following day. My situation was spinning out of control. And the spin would continue to accelerate.

*

Regaining consciousness the next day, I was watching ceiling tiles again as I returned to my hospital bed. I looked up to see Dr. Mankin, who may have said more than this, but what I remember was, "We may have to take the leg."

I learned that the infection was extensive. The donor bone was not living tissue and, said the orthopaedic fellow, "Bugs have that for lunch." He told me that when the surgical team saw the extent of my infection in the open wound, they spent a long time discussing what to do. They observed that the infection was moving into my host bone, the living parts into which the donor bone was grafted. All of the infected new parts were removed. Dr. Mankin did several things during surgery for the purpose of tightening the closure of the wound. A metal rod was inserted into my knee for some orthopaedic reason that I'm sure was very good. I had a fever. This was a serious infection and people die from such infections.

The pathology results indicated that three different bacterial organisms were cultured from my wound. I began intravenous antibiotics, two different medicines three times per day, in an isolation room. I learned that bacterial infection is toxic to cancer, in case any of that was present. *Tumor necrosis factor*, a previously unknown ally, was now a part of my vocabulary.

I also became aware of the pathology results from the tumor resection a month earlier, and there were mixed opinions regarding the news. My cancer diagnosis was determined to be *stage-3 angiosarcoma*. And there was a one-millimeter margin at one end of the tumor. The margin is the amount of surrounding healthy tissue that is excised with the tumor. A good margin would indicate that all of the tumor was removed. One of the orthopaedic fellows told me, "All we really need is a one-cell margin" to know that the cancer is gone. The cancer specialists were not so ebullient. I learned that *angiosarcoma*, a tumor made of blood vessels, could have a presence well outside of a surgical margin.

The pathology report went into additional disturbing details. The cancer cells were described as having "much mitochondrial activity." This was before Google, so I don't remember where I refreshed my understanding of mitochondria. But, yes, I remembered correctly from college biology: Mitochondria are the powerhouses of cells. And I recall the phrase "high grade malignancy" from the report. I have always been accustomed to doing things well. Apparently I can also grow some very good cancer cells. One oncologist gave me about a one in three chance of having a recurrence of the cancer.

I was recovering from a serious infection, my allograft was gone and in its place was a painful spike in my knee, and I wasn't out of the woods from an aggressive cancer. What else could possibly go wrong?

*

I had always known Dr. Mankin, my Gaucher specialist, to be a very dedicated, and hard working professional. I had observed it myself. I knew from my hospitalization during the prior month that he arrives at work long before sunrise. And, I saw him years earlier making rounds during the Eve of *Yom Kippur*. His command of the situation was a large source of my strength. I could not have foreseen that he himself would become seriously ill.

The information conveyed to me by the residents and fellows was that the doctor on whom I relied to make me better, was now himself a patient at the same hospital where I lay. I recalled my anesthesiologist's words, that by following Dr. Mankin's advice I would have my best chance for recovery. Now, he too was incapacitated.

On New Year's Eve my dinner tray included a serpentine blower-horn. It was a nice gesture from the Dietary Department. But it reminded me of the normal life outside of my current condition, a life that seemed so far away and receding. I was lonely and forlorn. I saw no alternative to pressing forward with a goal to recover. But my condition just continued to get more complicated with each new development. I was not feeling hopeless. But since that time I've often wondered, "Why was I *not* feeling hopeless?"

*

My parents were genuine, uncomplicated people. I was now a parent myself, and I felt their agony over seeing their child in bad condition. My mother commonly spoke from her heart, sometimes without running her words through a filter. She said what she meant. Years later, I used this example in my eulogy for her: "One day I said, 'Mom, do you like my new hat?' To which she responded, 'Oh, you're wearing a stupid, little hat.'" But when she expressed love, her message was similarly unrestrained and unedited. And in the isolation room where I now found myself in a state of disrepair and fighting a serious infection, my Mom said to me, "I don't know if this is even possible, but we're closely related. And if they can take a bone from my leg, you can have it." I have no doubt that she meant it. Live tissue donor bone transplantation was apparently not an option.

My leg was casted, from hip to toes, with a removable section to allow for dressing changes over the surgical wound. Hours before discharge from the hospital, a line was inserted through a vein in my arm to the entrance of my heart. I was brought to the Radiology Department to confirm proper placement of this central line. It was into this central catheter that I would give myself the six daily doses of powerful antibiotics. A nurse would come to my home every day to change the dressings over the surgical wound.

*

I sat in my den in a reclining chair, more miserable than ever. My knee was immobilized from inside with orthopaedic hardware, from the outside with the huge plaster cast, and everything hurt. I had reached a certain plateau in this episode and there was nothing else to do but sit, and presumably heal.

Sue took me to the orthopaedic clinic where I saw one of Dr. Mankin's associates. I was offered three alternatives. One plan would have them "clean up" the wound now, whatever that means, with a plan to attempt another allograft in a few months. Another option would be to take the fibula from my right leg, complete with its blood supply, and transplant it into the tibial position in my left leg. The third option would be to amputate the leg.

The surgical wound still looked very bad. In fact, it did not appear to be changing. This tissue had been irradiated, and so it did not have its full blood supply. And the area had been cut repeatedly and had most recently endured a serious infection. The most obvious conclusion was that this wound was not healing.

My wife brought me to see an oncologist near our home. We lived in a small town, and my oncologist was also a neighbor and a friend. He told us that *stage-3 angiosarcoma* has a fifteen percent five-year survival rate. He added that the first twenty-four months were the most critical. I had significant risk of cancer recurrence at the surgical site. And my lungs would need to be scanned regularly for any sign of metastasis. He said that a growth found in a lung could be excised as a wedge of lung tissue, and we could continue that procedure for every new spot, for as many times as necessary. Metastases could also erupt elsewhere in my body, and we would need to wait for that to happen before planning our response.

Together with the oncologist, Sue and I discussed the three options for the leg that were offered by the orthopaedists. I immediately rejected the idea of taking a bone from my healthy right leg. "We're not cutting into a healthy leg," I reasoned, "to try to save a leg that may be a lost cause." My oncologist, the friend and neighbor, was straightforward. "This is a very bad cancer," he informed us. He did not like hearing about a one-millimeter tumor margin. I recalled the pathologist's observation of "much mitochondrial activity." This *angiosarcoma* was playing for keeps. My intention was still to beat it. But I didn't know how much more of this I could take.

25.

Dr. Mankin, my trusted advisor and source of strength, was slowly resuming his work schedule. I called him by telephone. "I want your candid opinion," I said. I conveyed my conclusion that the idea of taking a live bone graft from my other leg was not an option. Another allograft meant that I would have surgery now, then heal for several months, if the wound healed at all, undergo the next grafting of bone, muscle, and skin, and then begin the lengthy rehabilitation. I would begin that rehabilitation only after the successful repeat of a procedure that didn't work the first time. And even if all of those components went according to plan, everything would change if the *angiosarcoma* reappeared.

The elephant lurking in the room was my Gaucher Disease. I wondered if my Gaucher bone would have sufficient growing power to remodel into and accept an allograft.

Pondering my dilemma, Dr. Mankin was briefly quiet. But then he was characteristically direct and unambiguous. "The prosthetics are very good," he said. He added, "People who elect for amputation have generally been quite pleased. Amputation is the fastest way back to work and your family." I thanked him and told him that I agreed. He put me in touch with the scheduler and a date was set for amputation surgery.

I called my parents. They would respect whatever decision I made, if I could tell them that this was also our trusted expert's recommendation. I didn't need to tell them that I had been through a lot. They too had been through a lot. "But," I said, "I need a better tumor margin."

26.

My father had been on the telephone with his friends at the Shriners Hospital, that landmark between my childhood home and my elementary school, where I had performed in high school for the "children in various stages of disrepair." I was invited to attend a teaching exercise in the amphitheater, known as the *Limb Deficiency Clinic*. Days before my scheduled amputation surgery, a surgery which I could cancel at any time, I accompanied my Dad into the Shriners Hospital.

I met with one of the prosthetists, the first such person in my life. The prosthetist accompanied us into the amphitheater, where I also met the chief of orthopaedic surgery, a physical therapist, and a nurse who was keeping everything organized. X-ray films were placed onto the light board, and I could see the bones of contorted limbs containing many metal parts. I saw images of limbs that ended abruptly, without the bones of legs or feet. Repeatedly, the side door would open and a smiling child would pull away from his parents, run toward the assembled adults and hop onto the examination table. To some children the orthopaedist would say, "Pop off your legs," and two legs would fall from the child and hit the floor with nearly simultaneous thuds. The orthopaedist, the physical therapist and the prosthetist expressed their observations and comments about what would need to be done next. Then, after being instructed, "Put your legs back on," the child would run into waiting parental arms and the family would exit. This was the routine, and it was organized and optimistic.

The biggest surprise to me was how bad the children's films looked, compared to how well they were moving. If I had seen only the pictures, I would have concluded that these were children who could not walk. Someone explained to me that these children are growing, so the prosthetist must keep up with them mechanically. It was an uplifting experience. I would keep my surgical appointment, as the next step in my complete recovery.

The prosthetist told me that, because the Shriners Hospital is a pediatric facility, they have experience with explaining these things simply. He offered to give me a short video to use for discussion of the issue with my children. We had a showing of *Hal Gets a Prosthesis* in the den with my children, the uplifting story of a Cabbage Patch Kid named Hal who had suffered a skiing accident.

*

I called my familiar anesthesiologist to see if she would be available for my surgery. But she and her husband were about to leave on a skiing trip. I admonished her to be careful and to not break a leg. She agreed that this was solid advice.

Sue brought me to Boston on a Sunday, with surgery scheduled for the next day. The oncology social worker joined us in my room. "What do we do," she asked rhetorically, "say goodbye to your leg?" I shrugged my shoulders. I no longer thought of the part inside the cast as "my leg." To me, it was something painfully sick that needed to be separated from the rest of me. I saw myself, minus the leg, as healthy.

The next day, my parents were present when a staff person arrived to wheel me to surgery. I assured my parents that I was completely at ease with my decision. In an area outside of the operating room I was met by people I presumed to be orthopaedic residents and fellows. They mentioned to me that the latest scans of my lungs were still clear, cancer free. I glanced around the room, looking for a telephone that I could use to call my family. I didn't see one. "Oh well," I thought, "I'll tell them later."

27.

I awoke to the sound of my name being loudly called from, it seemed, just inches away. There was a man somewhere below my waist, apparently very busy. I asked, "Are you the prosthetist?" He answered that he was, that I would go back to my room with a plaster cast, and that he would see me tomorrow.

I was conscious in the recovery room and I was pleased to accept the lollipop offered to me. I was aware of the other patients in this post-surgical area and thought that they all looked pretty bad. I asked for some extra lollipops because I knew that I would see my wife and older son in my room. He was due to be examined for the chronic fluid in his ears while I was in surgery.

I again watched ceiling tiles as I was wheeled to my room. My son greeted me. "Can I see your fake leg?" he asked. I said that I didn't have it yet, and handed him the lollipops from the recovery room. I resettled into my bed. I had an intravenous line in my left arm, an anesthetic line into my lower back, and I was comfortable.

*

I had no complaints during the evening, and I have just a vague memory of a nurse who was attentive and concerned for my comfort. Just after eleven o'clock that evening, as if timed to begin on the night shift, I began to have severe pain. The muscles in my thigh seemed to be in spasms. The contractions, if the muscles were indeed where this pain was originating, came intermittently and without warning. The pain was intense and seemed to elicit my involuntary screams. I called my nurse. Her response was that I was getting the full amount of medicine into the line in my back. I asked her to call the Pain Service. She refused. The spasms continued. I looked at the clock. It was midnight. I seemed to have no control of my voice and I screamed loudly. I called my nurse again. I asked her to call the Pain Service. She said, "They're all asleep." She assured me that I was getting enough medicine. This futile conversation continued for several hours. I was desperate. I didn't know what else to do. I have no memory of the time after about four o'clock. At about six o'clock in the morning I must have awakened. My nurse was standing next to me. She said, "You were asleep," in a manner that was exaggerated and perhaps slightly insolent. She seemed to me to be suggesting that I was, after all, sufficiently comfortable to sleep. I had fallen asleep, exhausted, after an agonizing, isolated, intensely painful night.

I am not aware of how, but my experience during the night seemed to be well known by the staff. A physician from the Pain Service came to my bedside. I said, "She wouldn't call you. She said you were all asleep." The Pain Service physician responded, "Maybe we were. But that's what we're here for." Some time that day, or maybe it was in the evening, a nurse came to my bedside. She said, "I heard what was happening last night. It was terrible."

During the day, a nicely dressed man with an overcoat over his left arm came into my room. In his right hand was a metal pipe connected to a flesh colored rubber foot. He pulled back my covering sheet and, with a satisfying click, the pipe with the rubber foot at its end was now an extension of my plaster cast. Then he covered me up again. With the words "I'll see you tomorrow," he turned and left.

That night, the same nurse who had refused to allow treatment of my pain, came into my room and greeted me in a friendly manner. Then she was gone and I never saw her again. I wondered how I could have been treated so callously by someone responsible for my care. "And," I wondered, "of all those people who seemed to have knowledge of what was happening to me, why didn't anyone take action to help me?" I thought that the treatment I received deserved to be reported to the appropriate health care accreditation and licensing agencies. But I just didn't have the energy left for another fight. I couldn't talk about this event for almost three years.

I have sometimes toyed with the idea of getting the nursing notes from that night, to learn the name of this deplorable person, this disgrace of a nurse. I would be interested to know her name and to discover if she is someone who managed to retain employment and her nursing license. But, no, I have done none of those things.

Why didn't the nurse who was later apologetic for the behavior of my nurse take some action herself? Was she afraid of bucking lines of authority? Was she afraid of making someone angry at her? I recalled the earlier occasion in my own professional life when I went along with the majority and then learned better. There is no substitute, nor is there any excuse, for a professional who does not adhere to the primary duty to care for the person entrusted to him or her. I recalled, "You're supposed to stand for something!" This experience radicalized me. I resolved to never serve a purpose other than the wellbeing of the person in my care, and to also fight for myself. These assertions would be tested.

*

I had some surgical pain in the area of my lower thigh, where my leg ended. But any surgical pain was overshadowed by the phantom pain. My foot hurt quite a lot. I could feel the pain in specific toes. Sometimes it seemed that a spike had been pounded into the side of my foot. Sometimes I felt a tickling sensation. I mentioned to my mother that my foot itched. I asked her to find the Pathology Department so she could scratch it for me. I was taking a very high dose of oral morphine, but the phantom pain was excruciating. It seemed to quiet at night and remained so for a few minutes after awakening. But for most of the day I was tormented by an aching part that did not exist.

Two days after amputation of my leg above the knee I was brought by wheelchair to the Physical Therapy Department. Carefully positioned between the bars, the prosthetist helped me up from the wheelchair. "You're standing," he said. I looked down to see two feet on the floor. He showed me how to wrap the residual limb. Providing compression would reduce the swelling, and would prepare the leg for casting of a prosthesis that would be capable of walking.

This would be a short inpatient hospitalization. I was home during the second week in February. I was done with the antibiotic infusions. And, without a huge cast, I was slightly more mobile with the crutches. I had the crude preliminary prosthesis from the hospital. The prosthetic socket was like a small barrel, into which I inserted my residual limb, held on with a wide belt that surrounded my waist. The rubber foot that I had first seen the day after surgery could be dressed with a sock and a shoe. It would be possible to dress in normal clothes and to go out.

28.

My birthday was less than three weeks away. I had been planning for this birthday. It was one of those milestone years and I had intended to celebrate. Now the celebration meant even more to me. I had picked the seats for a Wednesday matinee of *Phantom of the Opera* months before there was any sign of the bump on my shin that was the start of this whole episode. But I couldn't drive yet.

I chartered a limousine to pick up my wife and me to bring us to New York for the day. The boys would be with friends after school. To outward appearance I had two legs. But the temporary prosthesis from the hospital was not functional for walking, so I was again using crutches. We bought some things at the well-known *Zabar's* market, with our stretch limo and driver waiting outside. Then we went to *The Four Seasons* for lunch, and then our limo brought us to the theater. *Phantom* is one of my favorite shows. When the chandelier exploded and climbed to the ceiling during the prologue, I recalled all that had happened to me over the last six months, and I thought of how blessed I was to be able to see this again.

*

A different sort of phantom, the pain in a limb that no longer existed, was now my greatest misery. My high dose of daily morphine made me feel mentally fuzzy. An oncology psychiatrist informed me that phantom pain is similar to a small seizure occurring in the nerves that were cut. That seemed to make sense. She had me try several different current anticonvulsants, none of which did very much for me. My oncologist recommended an older drug that eventually worked quite well.

29.

Over a month had passed since my surgery and the time had come to start with a prosthetist. I had the first appointment of the afternoon with a prosthetist who was recommended to me by his colleagues at Shriners Hospital. He had once been the prosthetist in the operating room, I learned, in that role as the first person to begin the rebuilding of people awakening from amputation surgery. I also learned that the prosthetist was himself a lower extremity amputee. My father brought me to the office shortly after noon.

The prosthetist seemed to have a twinkle in his eye and an impish sense of humor. He asked, "What are your goals?" "That's easy," I said. "I want to go dancing, walk with a normal gait, and get back on my bicycle." There was a moment of silence before I asked, "Am I being realistic?" I cannot say for certain what words he used, but the reply I received was enthusiastically, emphatically affirmative. He added, "Orthopaedic surgeons think that amputation is a failure of their treatment. But for us it's just the beginning."

*

In the weeks that followed I learned much about the process of development of a prosthetic leg. And the prosthetist shared with me some of his personal details. He described returning to elementary school after his accident, with a wooden peg under him attached by a belt around his waist.

There was undisguised irritation in his voice as he quoted his third grade teacher: "You have to sit over here while the class plays. You're not like other children any more. You have to accept that." He said that at the time he thought, "Oh, yeah? Watch this." He was very matter-of-fact in this rebellious narrative. He did not seem to be trying to teach me something. But I had learned very well to discern the themes of a story while I was in my undergraduate course in modern fiction. That sophomore-level English literature class has served me well, personally as well as professionally in the science and art of personality assessment. I heard very clearly the theme of this narrative: The limitations are in the minds of everyone else. I don't need to accept them. And, invoking the existentialism of Jean Paul Sartre, which I also studied in that class, I understood that I don't need to live inside the compartments imposed upon me by others. You never know how a liberal arts education will be a benefit. And, for that matter, you never know how far is the reach of a third grade teacher.

My prosthetist informed me that my residual limb is very long and strong, with movement in all directions. I would have an effective lever, he told me, with which to control a new leg.

I told him about Gaucher Disease, and the well-established observation of an Erlenmeyer flask formation of the long bones of such people. My femur ended at the flair of the bone, creating a broad surface. I could see that he understood the physics and engineering of the device that he was about to build for me. And he was also building the mindset in me that would provide a foundation for the hardware.

The development of a leg is a complex undertaking, with casting of the residual limb, fabrication of a check-socket, adjustments to the check-socket to adapt to the changing biological tissues, and construction of the first model. My prosthetist said that public expectations became inflated following the television series *The Six Million Dollar Man,* with its quote in the opening credits, "We can make him better." We were just now, he told me, entering an age of high technology prostheses.

I attended physical therapy at a hospital. I walked in with crutches, wearing the temporary leg from the hospital. When the therapist asked me about my goals, I told her the same goals that I had told the prosthetist. She didn't seem to have a coherent idea of what to do with me. She advised me to get a wheelchair at the hospital entrance when coming for appointments. I had already been to the theater in New York, a local shopping mall and had walked to the Physical Therapy Department in my existing condition. I had no inclination to follow her advice to retreat to a condition of less independent mobility.

*

I did get some time on a stationary bicycle. But then the physical therapist seemed to think that I needed to know what to do if I were ever face down without a leg. So there I was, face down on a mat. "What's the first thing you do?" she asked. I didn't miss my cue. "I yell 'Help! I've fallen and I can't get up!'" I related this story to my parents by telephone, in an age when we still paid for long distance calls by the minute. It was a full twenty-five minutes of a long distance toll call before the three of us could stop laughing and catch our breath.

30.

The day arrived when I would be receiving my new leg. My Dad brought me to the prosthetist's office. The prosthetist carried the leg carefully into the room. He was being careful, not out of reverence. Rather, an unanticipated knee flexion could break the fingers of a person holding the leg without proper mindfulness. He showed me how to lubricate my residual limb to accept the custom socket. He explained that the four-bar design of the knee connected to its pneumatic piston would be stable enough to hold me vertically while standing, but would be sufficiently unstable to allow the knee to flex during the toe-off of my stride. During flexion the pneumatic piston would pressurize to then force the leg to extend as I stepped forward. It sounded very complicated.

I was sitting at the end of a walkway with parallel metal bars on either side. The prosthetist supervised my application of the suction socket. Then he told me to hold onto the bars with both hands and carefully stand. I looked down. I was vertical. I was standing on my own two feet.

The prosthetist, my instructor and role model for use of this new limb, didn't touch me physically, only with his words. "Move your leg forward and strike the heel to be sure that the knee is in full extension. Now move the weight of your body over the top of the leg and step forward with your right foot. Now bring your left foot forward and repeat the process." I was walking! I can walk!

When I reached the end of the walkway I turned and walked the other way toward him. He didn't make eye contact. The prosthetist's gaze was fixed upon the hardware, evaluating my gait. When I reached him, he put a hex wrench into a screw near the piston, gave it a slight turn and released me back into the walkway. I turned and walked away from him, then turned again toward him, then the other way. I was ecstatic. "I feel like I can run out of here," I told him.

I didn't look over to my Dad because I was afraid that I would fall if I didn't attend carefully to what I was doing. But I knew him well enough. I knew that he was in tears.

"I want you to beat the hell out of this," my prosthetist told me. "If you break it, I'll make you another one. But if you bring it back all shiny and clean, I'll know that you haven't been using it. This is a tool for you to use, for you to be a part of life."
"Can I go to the beach?" I asked.
"Go to the beach," said the prosthetist.
"What if I get sand in it?"
"You wipe it out," was the answer.
"What if I get it wet?"
"I've fallen out of a canoe with mine," said the high amputee who was told that he couldn't play like other children. I never heard the word "no" or the word "cannot" or the word "unable," in reference to himself or in reference to me. I was back. I was whole.

*

I found a different physical therapist. For one of my sessions we met at the bicycle shop. She helped to translate my needs to the bicycle mechanic. We found a mountain bike that could be configured with a quick-release on the shaft of the seat to allow me to get on and to then raise the seat under me. A large trap-style pedal on the left would keep my prosthetic foot attached and aligned. These pedals were only sold in pairs. I was eventually able to give the right pedal to someone with the same need as me on the other side.

I still fell down a lot when walking. I was keeping data, so I know that on some days I fell as many as six times. I was holding a cane for support. The standard advice of my physical therapists was to hold the cane in the contralateral hand. And because my left leg was the extremity with which we were currently involved, I was instructed to hold the cane in my right hand. But when I fell, it was because of unexpected flexion of the prosthetic knee on my left side. I was falling to my left. I threw out the professional recommendation, and started holding the cane in my left hand, where I needed the support. I stopped falling.

The phantom pain was becoming more manageable. I felt more normal without the morphine. I was never aware of any withdrawal symptoms. Since then I have met quite a few people who have been very sick while withdrawing from a lower dose of opiates than I had been taking. I have no explanation.

There are many tweaks and adjustments required for a new limb and I saw my prosthetist frequently. I enjoyed these meetings. Whatever mechanical issue I brought to the prosthetist was solved before I left. And his mental attitude was always optimistic and empowering. Humor was a large part of his life and he tried to keep serious matters in proper perspective. In that way he reminded me of my Gaucher doctor. On one such occasion my prosthetist told me that he wanted my need for a prosthetic leg to be inconvenient. I understood him. I replied, "As opposed to being totally disabling?" "Exactly," he said.

The latest technologies for prosthetic feet included energy storing designs, which could transfer the force of the heel strike to the toes, to assist with gait. They all looked like a rubber foot on the outside. The engineering was within. I would have the opportunity to try all of them.

I tested one that was similar to the design used by runners. I gave it back after a week of feeling catapulted down ramps. There was another model for me to try, whose rubber exterior would have been matched for someone with much darker skin than mine. I saw my prosthetist's mischievous twinkle when he suggested that maybe with this foot I would be able to play basketball.

Periodic scans of my lungs and examinations by my oncologist continued to show no evidence of cancer. By late spring I was back at my job in a psychiatric hospital. My life was in an ordinary routine. There was the absence of crisis.

31.

As predicted, the amputation option was the fastest way back to my family and work. At first I was falling less, and then I was not falling at all. I worried about the possibility of a recurrence of the cancer. But I was not hampered by this anxiety in everyday life. I seemed to be coping well.

Over the next couple of years I wondered *why* I was doing as well as I was. I spoke at a patient meeting that year. The group was shocked by my narrative. Some of the participants asked me about coping strategies. I told them what I had done that was comforting to me at the time. I recall speaking about how important it is "to allow yourself to cry." I was not being falsely modest when I related to the group how overwhelmed I felt at times. I noted how helpful it was for me to have people nearby who cared, and who allowed me to express my distress.

It was during this period of time that the Internet was becoming popular. I wondered if there could be a networked method of finding support. I found several support groups through the Internet. In at least one of them I heard, or rather, read statements that shocked me. I heard from people who were not coping well. And their descriptions of themselves and their situations seemed alien to my way of thinking.

I had considered my sick leg to be the repository of my sickness and distress. In this way of translating the situation to myself, I considered myself to be a healthy person — with a sick part. Removal of that sick part would allow the remainder of my body and psyche to continue on its healthy course. I was already well versed in an area of psychology known as *cognitive-behaviorism*. Cognitive-behavioral approaches in psychotherapy involve changes in thinking as well as changes in behavior.

People who are depressed may express some often-heard depressive thoughts, such as, "I'm worthless," "I'm hopeless," "I deserve to be miserable," "I should feel guilty for what has happened to me," and many more. Years earlier, I had attended a lecture by a psychologist well known in the field of cognitive-behavioral psychology. He summed up the depressive thinking of depressed people by saying, "They *kvetch*!" He then felt a need to define that word from Yiddish, the historical language of Ashkenazi Jews. Yiddish is a very emotionally expressive language, based upon what little I know of it. To *kvetch* means to whine or complain. And, in my New Englander's English version of the word, it can also be a noun, such as, "That whining and complaining person is such a *kvetch*."

As I looked for an online support group, I encountered people who conveyed some extremely unhelpful self-statements. I heard from a combat veteran who lost his leg in a land-mine explosion. He vividly described his mental imagery of the loss of his leg. He spoke of his leg as having died that day. He referred to that date as his first day of death. He was speaking of his body in the past tense, as if his demise was already preordained to occur in stages. I found his thinking to be foreign and disturbing. What is more important, he reported feeling depressed. He was not coping well. His self-descriptions of his situation were profoundly unhelpful to him. He seemed to be unaware of this point.

In these Internet discussions, I also encountered people who were in their homes, doing few, or no, activities that gave their lives joy or meaning. They spent their days *kvetching*. This is the behavioral part of cognitive-behaviorism. Their behaviors consisted of solitary activities, often without doing something that is recognizably pleasurable. Not surprisingly, social withdrawal and the absence of daily pleasure are part of the criteria for a diagnosis of depression. This impressed me as a tough way to live. They connected with people whose agenda was also *to kvetch* (infinitive), and their discussions with other *kvetchers* (noun) validated their life of *kvetching* (participle). And, as I said, these people were not coping well with their illnesses. This strategy was not healthy.

If the person's thinking connotes depression, and the person's behavior is that which is characteristic of depression, this would not seem to be a life that a person would choose, if that person's goal were to be happy. If all of these conditions were to exist, and there was no end in sight and no apparent solution, the emergence of hopelessness would be a logical result. Not surprisingly, hopelessness is one of the top two risk factors of suicidal behavior. Only a history of a prior suicide attempt is a greater risk factor. Hopelessness is second, ahead of depression.

I thought about my Thanksgiving Day holiday spent in excruciating pain. Suicide as a solution to my distress never occurred to me. I began to wonder, "Why not?" If ever I had a day in which my life was not worth living, that was it. So, why didn't I think about dying? It just never occurred to me.

I think that the difference between me and someone who may have become suicidal is that I always had a measure of hope. Sometimes my hope was strung along hour to hour by the Asian anesthesiologist. And it finally resulted in some measure of relief. In his attempt to be culturally aware and responsive, the anesthesiologist also gave me an orientation toward the future. Presumably, I would indeed be home for Hanukah.

Hearing my Asian anesthesiologist speak of Hanukah in his heavily accented English was mildly amusing. I was also enormously grateful for his very evident concern and attempt to relate to me. I felt connected with him, and I felt supported.

I recalled the imagery that I had invoked with regard to my cancer. It was a *Klingon Cruiser*. It was the *Wicked Witch of the West*. It was the *Uncircumcised Philistine*. In each of those images, I had the power to defeat it. I had the photon torpedoes. I had water. I had some small smooth stones. But, most importantly, I was reminding myself that my name includes *David,* a reference to the kid with the skill and courage to defeat the large enemy. I described my situation to myself in ways that invoked power, strength, and ultimate victory. I attributed to myself *health*, and I thought of myself as separate from the expendable part of me with the illness.

Another of the schools of existential thought that I learned in my sophomore modern fiction class was called *absurdism*. I never liked it very much, because it represented defeat in trying to understand what life is about. Those writers taught that we should stop trying to attach meaning to life, because it's all a crock. I had a lot of experience looking at ceiling tiles, either on the way to the operating room, or on the way back from the operating room. And I looked at ceiling tiles as I lay in my hospital beds, either waiting for a diagnosis, ruminating about a diagnosis, or just lying there without meaningful purpose. At those times, I thought about all of the important entries in my schedule that were too important to miss. Except that now I would miss them. I thought to myself, "This is the stupidest, the most absurd and meaningless thing that has ever happened to me." But my drive was to return home from the absurdist narrative and to once again find meaning.

I used humor to deflect the terror of the diagnosis and to stand back and look at the absurdity of my situation. One of my proudest moments in my cancer recovery story is when I exclaimed, "Help! I've fallen and I can't get up!" That, of course, was a quote from a television advertisement that was so hokey that it became an immediate cliché. This also has a psychological name. *Meta-cognition* is the activity of standing back and looking at the situation from a new perspective. It's a process of thinking about the thinking. And humor does that for me. Humor brings me to a place separate from my distress, where I can point to it and laugh at it.

*

The history of Ashkenazi Jews has often been wonderful, rich with joyful traditions. But the Ashkenazi history has also been tragic during the European experience. There are many examples of humor from the Holocaust, by which people in the deepest despair gained mastery over their oppressors.

When I was growing up, which involved many hours in front of a black and white television, one of the shows I watched was a comedy set during World War II. Interestingly, at least two members of the cast were themselves Ashkenazi Jews from Europe. My understanding is that at least one actor agreed to perform only if he were allowed to portray his Nazi character as a fool. One of my favorite jokes is the history of the Jews in less than a second: "They tried to kill us; we won; let's eat." We always win when we can laugh at the enemy.

I come from this tradition of using humor to deflect pain. My grandfather, the only member of his family to come to America before the Holocaust, and thus, the only survivor, had a wry sense of humor. I believe that he deflected horrible psychological pain, especially when the fate of the Jews of his hometown became known. I'm not aware if humor, like

Gaucher Disease, is inherited. But if humor is not genetic, I had twelve years to pick it up from my grandfather.

*

In the first few years following my cancer recovery, I was working and also trying to stay current with the latest psychological research. I, and a few dozen colleagues in southeastern Connecticut sometimes met for an educational seminar at one of the local colleges. On one such occasion, a psychologist was due to present a lecture entitled *Group Therapy in Breast Cancer Treatment*. Those of us in the lecture hall were ready to politely listen to this woman's professional experience and results. We anticipated hearing about the palliative efforts of the mental health staff with their distressed patients.

What we received was much more. The data presented by the psychologist showed predictions of greater durations of survival of the cancer patients, based upon their emotional responses. This was jaw-dropping news. Psychologists were unaccustomed, at least in those days, of hearing that their efforts actually saved the lives of cancer patients. We knew we could help people to feel better. Hearing that we could also help cancer patients to live longer was more than we expected.

The psychologist reported that, based upon the categories of responses by the patients to some seemingly ordinary therapeutic activities, she could predict how long they would live. She had data showing that certain cognitive responses were related to statistically significantly longer life spans.

We always need to be cautious about assuming that a variable related to another variable is causing the change. Remember, tall men are associated with purchases of long trousers, but we cannot make men taller by lengthening their clothing.

Perhaps this could be different. If certain psychological responses can be shown to be associated with survival, then psychologists are especially good at conditioning behaviors. We may be able to save lives.

The psychologist reported that her patients were instructed to draw pictures of their cancers. Then, the patients were instructed to perform some action upon their cancers in their pictures. The patients' drawings and verbal responses fell into four categories. There were some patients who were stoic in their drawn narratives. Some patients showed that they felt defeated. Other patients were angry at their cancers. And still other patients seemed to be denying that they had cancer.

Part of the results that the psychologist presented were surprising. "Denial has not been considered to be a good thing, historically, in psychology," she said. But the patients who were "in denial" were among those who survived best. Perhaps "denial" was not the best descriptor for what was going on with these patients. They were not depriving themselves of treatment. And they were not denying, as in being oblivious to, their cancer. Rather, they were compartmentalizing their illness and going on with the rest of their lives. Such a patient's internal dialogue may be something like, "Yeah, yeah, I know about this cancer stuff. But I have my granddaughter's graduation to go to in a month and I'm going to be there."

The angry patients also did well. They were not angry with themselves or with the people around them. They were angry at the cancer, and at the ridiculously absurd state of affairs in which they found themselves. This response most closely reminded me of what I had been thinking, a strategy that seemed to have worked well for me.

The patients whose responses placed them in the categories of stoic or defeated did not do as well, based on the data of a large sample of people.

I felt that I had found part of the answer to what had helped me to survive. I recalled feeling frustrated and angry. I had imagery in my head of power and victory. I used humor to deflect emotional pain. I attributed the concept of health to myself overall, while acknowledging that my leg was sick and had to go. I had the emotional support of people around me. I had hope.

My cancer started in a bone lesion related to my Gaucher Disease. To my relief I was now receiving infusions of a medicine for Gaucher Disease, the underlying cause of everything I had been through. I was hopeful. I had good reason to anticipate a healthy future. I sat in my oncologist's chemotherapy room with people who were suffering greatly, some with limited life expectancies. I saw some of the emotional responses that were reported in the research I learned about in the seminar. I wanted to psychologically support some of the clearly defeated people I encountered. But my role there was limited to that of a casual, if friendly, acquaintance. I was there to be a patient in the chemotherapy room, not a psychologist.

32.

I thought of the role of social connectedness in dealing with depression. I thought of the role of social support in maintaining hopefulness. And I thought of the potential role of a socially charitable purpose to provide me with a tax deduction for my Internet involvement. In 1994 we still had to pay a monthly fee for a slow connection to the Internet over a telephone line. I didn't like the idea of another utility payment.

During my infusions in the oncologist's chemotherapy room, people with active malignancies surrounded me. I still wasn't sure what the Internet was, so I used the time available to me during my infusions to read. I learned about the needs that led to the design of the early Internet. As a headless, indestructible communication system arising from military strategic planning during the Cold War, the Internet was designed to be simultaneously compatible with all of the different types of hardware that are connected to the network. I wanted a Gaucher Disease network to also be compatible with whatever hardware a person used, no matter how unsophisticated. Some people may have office computers. Others may have computers at home. And I had heard of cell phones that, incredibly to me at the time, could receive emails. The computer that I myself had at home had a fraction of the number-crunching power of the computer I would someday carry in my pocket. The idea of a powerful microprocessor that would control the gait components of a bionic leg was still a science nerd's fantasy.

I found an online service that was devoted to Jewish causes. I proposed to them a discussion group dealing with Gaucher Disease. No one in this Internet service devoted to Jewish causes had ever heard of Gaucher Disease. They had heard, however, of Tay Sachs Disease. So I told them, "Gaucher is in the group of diseases that includes Tay Sachs. Gaucher Disease is twice as prevalent as the disease you've heard of, but it's different." They consented to create the discussion group, if I agreed to include all of the diseases that are at increased frequency within Jewish populations.

Gaucher Disease now had an Internet presence. But I wasn't entirely clear what had been created. I expected to find an online bulletin board, a device which people called a *web log*. Some time later the colloquial usage was shortened to *blog*. To my surprise, what had been created was an email distribution list. But to be universally compatible with a wide range of hardware types, the Gaucher Disease group would need to be a text-only discussion. In those days computer viruses were also an issue, and text prevented exposure to that risk.

This became useful to an increasing number of people concerned with Gaucher Disease and related disorders. The group has migrated to several different host systems over its history. It remains today as a gathering of hundreds of people with a common interest in Gaucher Disease.

I had set up a website, rudimentary by today's standards, devoted to Gaucher Disease. I put a hit-counter on the bottom of the homepage to record how many times the page was viewed. One week, much to my surprise, the number on the hit-counter began to increase by thousands each day. I assumed that there was some sort of malfunction. But then I discovered that my page, apparently selected randomly, was featured that week on one of the *Yahoo!* system's web pages.

I started to receive email from strangers. Some people asked innocent questions. A couple of people accused me of being a Nazi, apparently because I used the words "Jewish" and "genetic" in the same paragraph.

One person wrote to express his relief that he now had an explanation for his chronic weight problem. He concluded that with his Ashkenazi heritage, and the knowledge that Gaucher Disease is a disorder of lipid storage, he has the answer he had been seeking. I reluctantly informed him that the total amount of *glucocerebroside* stored within the body of a person with Gaucher Disease is extremely small. Obesity is a totally different sort of lipid storage disorder.

*

A meeting of the National Gaucher Foundation was due to be held in late 1994 in Philadelphia. I looked forward to reconnecting with old friends and hearing the news about our treatment. In the evening we had dinner in a large hotel ballroom. I spotted Abby and her mother. Both were looking happy and healthy. We sat together at a round table. Abby sat immediately to my right. Abby was now fourteen years old, and was still receiving regular intravenous infusions of our missing enzyme. Her episodes of bone pain were less frequent. Abby was aware that another bone crisis could occur without warning, at any moment. But on this evening she was free of pain and she could see the possibility of a healthy future without the devastatingly painful episodes.

There was some sort of music playing, surely quiet enough to allow people to talk comfortably. During a lull in our conversation, Abby turned to me and without warning asked, "Can I have my dance now?" My throat closed up and I think my heart may have skipped a beat. We stood up next to our table, and I wrapped my arms around her. I recalled all that had happened to me since the telephone conversation from my hospital bed. Abby had remembered the promise, and now the commitment was met.

33.

In my life as a psychologist I gravitated toward work of ever-increasing intensity. I had long since left public schools and was devoted to work within institutional settings. I felt a kinship with people excluded from everyday life by disabling conditions. I rarely discussed my own experiences, but that strand of my life was never far from my consciousness.

I was a psychologist in a psychiatric hospital. My patient population had hospitalizations of very long durations. I would occasionally find myself in other parts of the large campus, including units with patients who would be in the facility for most of their lives.

Very often I was responsible for providing expert testimony at hearings of the Probate Court. There the issues involved involuntary retention in the hospital, or even, rarely, the involuntary administration of medication. I always thought of this duty as a very serious responsibility, with a huge potential for coercion and misuse. Involuntary hospitalization, commonly referred to as *commitment*, was legally justifiable only on the basis of extreme danger to self, danger to others, or on the basis of grave mental disability.

The security of my unit was prudent, but not overly restrictive. Prior to the hearings pertaining to my patients, I would often witness the hearings of patients from a very high security unit. A patient would be led by one or two uniformed security officers, hands shackled to a waist belt. The patient would sometimes read a prepared statement, hands trembling, imploring the judge to make this the annual review that would result in discharge to freedom. Members of the patient's professional team would also speak, describing the patient's current functioning, and perhaps referencing the history of horrible events that led to the patient's referral to a high security mental hospital. I rarely saw a patient dismissed from hospitalization at one of these hearings. Most often the patient would be led from the room by the uniformed officers, in shackles and tears.

I thought of how these patients' behavioral histories paralleled my history of Gaucher Disease symptoms. Patients such as these pose a vexing treatment problem, with histories of problem behaviors that are of very high intensity, but very low frequency. There are murderers in that population who don't kill very often. Similarly, I have had comparatively few Gaucher Disease problems when I consider my history year to year. Severe bleeding, bone crises, bone infarctions, cancer, and infection can be life changing and life threatening. But they don't happen very often.

At one court hearing, I was very aggressively examined by the attorney representing my patient. He made me justify every statement, and every assertion. If we were going to prevent his client from re-entering everyday life, I would need to prove, to the required legal standard, that the safety of the client or the safety of others required restrictive measures. I took this responsibility seriously. I was prepared for my testimony with documentation of firsthand behavioral observations and reliable frequency data of serious target behaviors.

I believed in my professional judgment. And I believed in my good intentions. But I also had experience as the person dependent upon others for my care, or for my life. I had unquestioning trust in my orthopaedic anesthesiologist prior to my cancer surgery. I believed her when she said that she would watch over me during surgery and keep me from harm. Now I, too, had the responsibility to stand for something.

I also believed in a system that doesn't give one person, no matter how well intentioned, the power to incarcerate someone or to force chemicals into another person's body. Anyone asking my parents would certainly hear that I was a great psychologist. But if my opinion were to prevail at this hearing, I would want that judgment to be based upon the weight of the evidence I presented. I intended to stand for something. I expected the patient's attorney to make me prove my case. I was relieved that he did.

The judge ruled in favor of continued hospitalization of our patient. Shortly afterward, I found myself in the elevator with the attorney who had questioned me so aggressively. He looked down and said nothing. He looked very uncomfortable. I told him that he had done a good job. And I meant it.

*

I had a patient with a very bad cancer. I and a staff person brought him to his doctors' appointments. He would need some combination of surgery and radiation. I knew from my own experience how this would mean a period of extreme unpleasantness. I found this patient to be a very endearing person. I felt a great deal of empathy for him. I felt that I understood some of his challenges.

Unlike my own situation years before, radiation and surgery were not sufficient to halt his malignancy. His cancer metastasized and his life expectancy was short. I met the oncologist at the entrance to the patient's room in the Intensive Care Unit of the general hospital. The oncologist described the prognosis as "grim." Two of the patient's family members were present and they briefly described the funeral plans.

I entered my patient's room and stood on the side of his bed. My patient looked up at me with wide eyes. I could see on the monitor that his blood pressure was extremely low. He was too weak to move or to talk. I grasped his right hand in my hands. I spoke to my patient. I don't recall what I said to him but, not knowing the status of his cognitive processes, I know that I was trying to speak slowly. There was no outward response from the patient, and I saw no evidence of distress. I cannot say what, if anything, he understood of my visit. But he seemed to be aware of my presence.

I returned to my facility and to the psychiatric unit whose census listed this patient as admitted, but currently absent. This patient's chart was still in the nursing office. He would be our patient until he returned, or until his demise at the general hospital. I briefly pondered what my responsibility might be at this moment.

I was still his psychologist and I had interacted with him in a professional capacity. I concluded that I had a responsibility to write a progress note pertaining to my interaction that day with my patient. I wouldn't have very much to say. The patient was dying and had very little strength. I wrote that the patient appeared to be comfortable and that there was no outward indication that he was in pain.

Not long after my patient's death, I was summoned by the psychologist responsible for my professional performance reviews. He informed me that a complaint had been filed against me for unprofessional behavior. I learned that a nurse had taken offense at my progress note referencing my patient's pain level. Her contention was that pain is assessed by nurses, not by psychologists, and that I had acted outside of the scope of my profession.

I recalled the nurse in New York many years earlier who casually asked, "What's the emergency?" in response to my pain. My thoughts also turned to the night following my amputation and how not a single nursing professional who was aware of my situation would address my extreme pain. And I recalled my oath to myself that no one in my care would ever be treated like that.

I went to the office of my manager, who was already aware of the complaint. I knew this manager, whose profession also happened to be nursing, to be a person of great integrity and compassion. I demanded a copy of the complaint. I think she could see that I was understating my anger. She said that the form was somewhere in her office and that she would find it for me.

I have little doubt that my manager had already placed the complaint where it deserved to be and, as the saying goes, flushed twice. I always remained polite in my interactions with the nurse who found fault with my assurance that our mutual patient was comfortable. But I didn't extend myself beyond the requirements of social propriety.

*

On one warm, sunny, late-summer day in the second week of September, 2001, the news on television was of a major terrorist attack in New York, near where I had participated in a bicycling event, and not too far from where I was working. Our buildings were locked and we would stay in the residential unit for the near future. I expected that we would be receiving patients from other hospitals, especially if space was needed in community hospitals for physical trauma cases arriving from New York.

Our patients, a population which our legal system judged to be too dangerous to freely walk the streets, seemed childlike, scared, and vulnerable. That day I realized that terrorism is psychological warfare. And I was expected to treat patients for the same trauma that was affecting me.

By the end of the day we learned that there were few, if any, survivors of physical trauma being evacuated from New York. The dimensions of the psychological trauma were not yet evident.

I had seen the movie *Gettysburg* years earlier. This is the sort of story that I expected to learn in the course in military science at Alfred University during my exceedingly short military career. I was inspired by one character, also a New Englander, who taught college English before becoming a leader in battle. Anticipating a charge by the enemy he says in the film, "Let's see how professors fight." I checked with the historical society devoted to him, and apparently that line was written just for the screenplay. There is no evidence that Joshua Chamberlain, English professor and recipient of the Congressional Medal of Honor ever actually said that. But I found the statement to be inspiring nevertheless. The battlefields in the new century would be psychological, a domain in which I was now skilled and experienced. I would make a contribution to my country, without ever shining a button or marching in a straight line.

I and many of my colleagues volunteered in a variety of different ways. We said, "We're psychologists, collectively with a zillion years of education, and this is psychological trauma. Where are we needed?" Some of my colleagues were already on disaster teams. I and many others joined training classes in preparation for deployment to service centers.

One of my colleagues went out first. We had our pick of locations. She decided to deploy to a service center in lower Manhattan, close to Ground Zero. We were already hearing about a strange respiratory irritation that was affecting responders in that area. I was aware that lung problems could occur with Gaucher Disease. I decided that I didn't need any additional medical complications.

I deployed to a call center that was focused mainly upon the needs in New York, but located hundreds of miles away. The casework was intensely emotional. I was called upon to provide cultural interpretation on a couple of occasions, as mental health people encountered the religious Jewish communities in New York.

I thought that I was comfortable with the emotional trauma to which I was exposed for eight hours each day. We were warned of vicarious traumatization, sometimes called caregivers' stress, but I ignored the advice. During the weeks after my return home, I continued to receive mailings containing advice to make contact with my colleagues. I thought, "I'm a psychologist. I know how to handle my stress." I threw the literature into the trash.

A few months later I was asked to give a talk to a community group that was interested in what I had done in our country's disaster mental health response. I reached a point in my lecture where I casually related how I felt one day while I was debriefing someone's extremely emotional circumstances. I heard the words leave my mouth, the first time I had spoken of this aloud. My throat closed. I couldn't breathe. I couldn't talk. I thought, "Oh my God. I'm going to cry in front of all these people." I took deep breaths. I recovered. I finished my presentation. But never again did I conclude that, just because I am personally familiar with emotional intensity, am I immune from psychological trauma.

*

I was nevertheless drawn to high intensity work. I began to moonlight as an Emergency Department psychologist. The chief psychologist informed me, "People either love this work or hate it. There appears to be no in-between." He was right. I saw colleagues become overwhelmed and decide to work elsewhere. At times I could see why they hated it. But even though each shift was stressful, often in unforeseeable ways, I felt a strange compulsion to return. Maybe it was the special camaraderie among emergency workers. Maybe it was the stimulation from handling situations that were at the peak of acuity. Maybe it was the challenge of applying intellectual rigor to figure out complex situations correctly. Or perhaps it was the special satisfaction known to people who can help others when they need it the most. I believe it's all of those factors. I felt that I had a duty to be in that place, if I had the stomach for it, because few people have the ability and the fortitude. I thought that perhaps the intense events I had endured in my own life were indeed a part of my *curriculum vitae*, my "plan of study of life."

34.

My early experience with incorrect diagnoses is apparently not unusual within the Gaucher community. Gaucher Disease simply does not have sufficient prevalence to cause physicians to readily consider it as a likely diagnosis, even for children with the symptoms that I evidenced very early.

Attempting to address this educational need, Dr. Pramod K. Mistry asked me to participate as a guest lecturer for a class at Yale Medical School for the first time in 2004. The plan was for him to begin the class, tracing Gaucher Disease from its molecular chemistry, through its genetics, and its effect upon the various body systems. This was a huge quantity of information to impart in a half hour. Then the plan was for me to speak for an hour, relating the disease's effects upon my health, and a global view of the effect of the disorder upon my life.

I prepared a few graphics to use for my lecture. I decided to use humor liberally, because I wasn't sure how interested the students would be. I decided to list my symptoms in chronological order, which seemed appropriate for an audience of future diagnosticians. I started with my first indication of a large spleen, the nosebleeds, the false diagnosis of mononucleosis, and all the rest of the narrative. When I got to 1993 in my list, I stopped to think. What was my next symptom? What was the next bad event attributable to Gaucher Disease? Bleeding, infection, bone crisis, infarction, fatigue? Anything? What about cancer? A little nosebleed, perhaps? Nothing. I couldn't think of one new manifestation of Gaucher Disease that has troubled me since 1993. That was the year that I began biweekly infusions of my missing enzyme. My list of symptoms simply came to an end with the beginning of enzyme replacement therapy. This was extraordinary news. And the point was not lost on the students, many of whom swarmed around me after the class to thank me and to discuss the issues further.

*

The two strands of my life, the Gaucher Disease narrative and the Everything Else story, started to unexpectedly intertwine. One day in a hospital Emergency Department, I intentionally "outed" myself to save someone's life.

It was several days before another planned lecture for the medical students. I had just finished evaluating a case and I was sitting at my workstation dictating the report into the telephone. Using my workstation's telephone to dictate my report meant that I would not be interrupted by an incoming call. I never learned how to pause the recording and, besides, I need to focus completely on what I'm saying. I take the quality of my diagnostic report very seriously. I'm supposed to stand for something, or some such internal directive. I don't want to be interrupted.

I became aware of one of the emergency physicians and a nurse hanging over me. I tried to ignore them as I continued to talk into the phone. But when I glanced up, they saw an opportunity to grab my attention.

"We need a stat psych consult," blurted the physician.

I am very happy to hear that my work is indispensable. But, really? Is the opinion of the psychologist so necessary that it deserves *drop-everything-and-do-this* status? The ER doc was not leaving until he had my full attention. I hung up the phone in the middle of my dictation. I knew that the last line of my report would be a note from the transcriptionist saying, "Dictation ended abruptly." I would need to fix the report later.

This was a hospital Emergency Department, so it was not entirely inappropriate for me to invoke the same words as that insensitive nurse in New York following my surgery after high school. "What's the emergency?" I inquired.

The physician described a situation involving a young man. He was a mostly healthy young adult. But he had an acute problem that needed immediate medical treatment. This was a problem that the young man had survived before. I was told that he had several hours to live, unless he had the necessary treatment. The problem was that he was refusing to be treated.

I've worked in settings where people can be legitimately judged to be incapable of making an informed decision. The mechanism within the long-term settings is to convene a Probate Court hearing immediately, and let the judge make the decision. But in this case, the young man seemed to be fully aware of his situation. And time was very important. He had no mental health treatment history and the emergency physician's opinion was that the patient had the mental competency necessary to legally refuse treatment. The ER doc wanted to know if I agreed.

I entered the patient's room and he politely offered his right hand to me when I introduced myself. I worked some questions pertaining to orientation into the conversation. The patient appeared to be fully oriented to his surroundings and to his situation. He understood that he would die soon without treatment.

"What do they want to do to you?" I asked him.

"They have a list of things they want to do to me," he said.

"What did they say would happen to you without treatment?" I inquired.

"They said I will die," he answered matter-of-factly.

"And you're OK with that?" I asked.

"Yup," was the answer.

We chatted for a while. The patient appeared to be mentally competent. I mentally listed the possible suicidal risk factors that I could assess during an interview. I found no evidence to legitimately allow me to say that he was intentionally self-destructive.

I said, "Let me make sure I understand this. You want today's date to be on your gravestone."

"I'm comfortable with that," he replied.

I decided to change the subject.

"Do you have a will?" I asked.

"I don't own anything," said the patient.

"Everybody has *something*," I gently disagreed. "Those disgusting socks belong to you," I added. He laughed appropriately at my stupid attempt at humor.

"What does your family think?" I asked him.

"They don't like it," he said, "but I just don't want to live like this, having the same problem and having to get treated again and again."

I asked him what it is about the hospital experience that makes it so unpleasant. He said, "I don't like needles." I reminded him that the physician had offered to give him medicine for anxiety, and that he would be prevented at all times from being in pain. An anesthetic could numb the site of any injection. Similar to the medicine I received prior to very aggressive surgery on my leg, he could have medicine so that he would feel comfortable and relaxed. "And," I added, "because you don't abuse these drugs, which could make giving them to you a bad idea, they'll break out the really good stuff for you."

"I just don't think that this is a life," he said, "coming to the hospital, getting better, and then having it happen again." The patient was not moved by my promise of comforting medicine and of a pain-free experience. He was content to let his recurrent problem follow its natural course and then to let this be the last day of his life.

I come from a cultural tradition that has sayings such as "Choose life," and "Where there is life there is hope." I've learned from my own experiences that I have a personal bias against death. I know what losing consciousness from a potentially mortal condition feels like. I remember feeling frustrated and angry at that moment. I have been able to demonstrate and confirm to myself my own valuing of life. I have tenaciously clung to my own life. Even on my most desperate day following the allograft, dying never occurred to me as a way out of my predicament.

Perhaps my beliefs about the value of life grow from my cultural upbringing. Or perhaps my beliefs valuing life are just a part of my personal makeup. Whatever the reason, I was not personally comfortable with seeing this mostly healthy young man allow his own preventable death.

I also gave some consideration to my recollection of a professor somewhere in the past who admonished my class of almost-psychologists to remain client-centered at all times. A professional discussion is not about us, it's about the person we are trying to help. My professional obligation is to respect the choices of the individual in my care. This, however, was a conundrum not anticipated during my university education.

I could not think of another line of questioning to explore with this young man, to try to identify some reasoning that I could gently disprove as a good cognitive therapist. I agreed with the emergency physician that there was no mental impairment to justify our involuntary treatment of him.

For me, however, fighting for life, or even just fighting for health, is personal. "Oh well," I thought. "I've got nothing else." So I sat back, looked the patient in the eye and said, "I have a disorder that makes me have an IV every other week."
"You?" He was incredulous.
"Yes," I said, "I get an intravenous infusion every other week. And I have lots of blood tests. It's what I have to do to stay alive. Personally, I accept it as a life. I'm OK with it."

He listened attentively. But then he seemed to retreat and said, "Yeah, well, that's not for me." And with that, I thanked him for talking to me, wished him well, and left the room. I told the emergency physician that our patient was still refusing treatment, and that I thought that he was mentally competent to make that decision. We could not force him to live.

I returned to my workstation. I logged in to my dictation account to see if the interrupted report was there yet. Before I could find the report, the emergency physician was standing over me again. "He has agreed to treatment," he told me. Perhaps I had an effect as a coping role model, a person of some responsibility in an Emergency Department, who yet endures needles. But I cannot be certain of his motivation.

I wanted to know what had changed his mind. But my involvement with this case was finished. I wouldn't want to say something that could possibly alter the outcome. Any further conversation with him would be for the purpose of satisfying my own curiosity, and not for the patient's wellbeing. When I next walked past the room where I had seen the young man, he was already gone from the Emergency Department, having signed consent for transfer to elsewhere in the hospital, for the procedures that would save his life.

I related this story from the Emergency Department the following week at a lecture to the medical students. I used this as an example of a good outcome that was only possible because I had survived everything that had happened to me.

*

Paraphrasing the advice that Mrs. Gump gave to Forrest, the practice of emergency services is like a box of chocolates. You never know what you're going to get. Patients are sent to the Emergency Department often for dangerousness, or for behavior that is unusual. And sometimes patients refer themselves when they are aware of being in great distress. But as I told that insensitive orthopaedic resident back in Boston, "They're all important."

I always expect that there will be much more to a story than its surface details. In my experience, an initial complaint that is stated vaguely has sometimes meant that someone is trying to escape from a bad situation. Sometimes a patient is relieved to finally be alone with a caring professional, someone expected to respond appropriately to distressing or even dangerous circumstances.

On one occasion years earlier, a registration clerk urgently brought to me the form containing a patient's consent for treatment. Under the wife's signature was the message, "He's beating me." A person reaching out for my help deserves the appropriate professional response warranted by the situation. I was always prepared to assertively maintain control of the emergency assessment to properly assess and treat and, if necessary, protect the person in my care.

On one busy evening, a woman presented herself, accompanied by her husband, to the Emergency Department with a vague complaint of anxiety. The patient asked to meet with me with her husband present. I was careful to ensure that this new patient really did want the attendance of her spouse.

Upon meeting this woman, I was pleasantly surprised to be able to rule out the worst of the possibilities. I sat with the patient and her very supportive husband in a private area. The woman seemed to be very uncomfortable. She reported to me that during the day she and her husband were at a local shopping mall. She met an acquaintance there, and stopped to talk. During this conversation with her friend in a public setting, she then had a sudden, unexpected, and very large bowel accident.

"That's humiliating," I said, apparently achieving the accurate empathy that makes me a good psychologist.

She was grateful for the understanding, and even more grateful when I offered to ask the emergency physician for medicine for her anxiety. She seemed to be partially calmed by this debriefing of the day's socially traumatic event. I left the patient in the room with her husband, so that I could talk to the physician.

When I returned, the patient appeared to be distressed again. Apparently, while she and I conversed eye-to-eye, her husband was able to get a good look at me. And he had a chance to talk with his wife while I was out of the room. My prosthetic leg at the time did not have a cosmetic covering. My cuffed, business-casual khakis rode up just enough at the ankle to reveal an aircraft-grade aluminum pylon. The patient said to me, "I know you've had some serious problems. And here I am complaining about my pissant issue." I reiterated that nothing diminished the seriousness of what had happened to her. I felt bad that I had unintentionally trumped her distress.

*

I had no such reluctance, however, when my needs exceeded those of another. I had already been radicalized by my contact with people who fell short of adherence to the responsibility of their professions. I recalled the nurse in New York who was dismissive of my post surgical pain, the orthopaedic resident who considered my distress to be that of one of many bothersome patients, the night nurse who refused to address my post amputation pain, the other night nurse who was aware of my distress and took no action, and even a co-worker who confronted my concern for the pain of someone else.

The vast majority of the professionals who have ever been responsible for me, and the vast majority of providers who have worked with me in our responsibility to others, have been fine people and superlative professionals. But I had resolved to assertively adhere to my own values, independent of anyone else's example or opinion. Never again would I be reticent during development of a treatment plan in which I could not have full confidence. Never again would I remain reticent while someone else was abused by a self-serving credentialed professional. Never again would I allow someone who should know better, give less than what a professional owes. I would expect professionals to stand for the principles of their professions, and I would demand the same of myself. I would stand for something.

I shared my commute to work in a van with a half dozen others who worked at the same facility. I found riding in a van to be unbearably boring. I enjoyed the ride and the conversations with my colleagues more when I was approved to be a driver.

One of my passengers was very anxious one day, as we traveled home during a heavy snowfall. I reassured her by saying, "I went to college near Buffalo," as if that's a part of my academic credentials for driving in winter. She was indeed reassured and we arrived home safely.

Everyone on the van was thrilled to discover that with me as driver, they also had the benefit of a handicapped parking space close to the building. They didn't know previously that I was walking on a right titanium hip and a left prosthetic leg. When they asked me how I obtained a special parking permit, I told them that the parking privilege usually costs an arm and a leg, but that I got a discount.

I do not always use the preferential parking privileges that come with having just one leg. But sometimes a skin abrasion can make walking with the prosthesis painful. And at other times, especially in New England, an icy pavement can make walking treacherous for me. It is possible for me to fall down with my left leg prosthesis even on dry pavement. But on ice, with only one foot that can feel its position, I am at increased risk. And I am very conscious of the danger that a twisting fall can pose to the implanted titanium hip on my right side.

In late winter, temperatures in New England can be above the freezing point during the day, only to fall well below freezing at night. The result is a melting of snow and ice that becomes a thin ice covering before morning. Weather forecasters commonly refer to this as black ice, because the thin coating on walking and driving surfaces cannot be easily seen.

On one such morning I piloted the van to the parking area. All of the handicapped parking spaces were occupied, one by an administrator who was standing near her vehicle with a member of her staff. I stopped the van, and hopped down.

"May I have that spot?" I asked.
The immediate response I received was, "Why do you need it?"

The short answer in my mind was, "Because I am legally entitled to it and you are not." And I was aware of a much longer answer which would have been a recitation of my orthopaedic history, and the legislature's rationale for establishing preferential parking for people with an established need, and my view that a professional needs to respect the law while on the job. But I was not so pleasantly instructive. I was outraged that I needed to justify my legal use of a designated handicapped parking space to someone who was using it for her personal convenience. I'm certain that I told her that she was rude and in violation of the law. It was ugly.

She yelled to her subordinate, "Call our police!" *Our* police indeed. I told her again that she was rude adding, "You don't make up your own laws!" I expected this professional to stand for something.

She did move her vehicle from the handicapped space. I used a cane to stabilize my gait on the icy pavement as I made for the door, turning at least once to reiterate to her that she was quite wrong.

Arriving in my office I picked up the telephone and called the security department. "This is Doctor Rosenfield. Are you looking for me?" I demanded. The stunned officer responded, "Uh, n-no, sir. We're not interested in getting in the middle of arguments over parking spaces."

Some time later, a nursing colleague mentioned to me that my name came up during a meeting. I'm not fully aware of the context, only that I was referred to as "That loudmouth Jew." I rarely have confrontations such as the parking lot incident, so there was likely a connection.

I pondered whether this obviously pejorative public reference to me required my response. I asked myself, "What is a loudmouth?" I concluded that a loudmouth is someone who makes you hear his opinion, even when you don't want to hear it. And then I asked myself, "What is a Jew?" To that I concluded that I certainly define and openly describe myself as one. I characterize myself as a member of the group whose values form the moral basis of Western Civilization, and if I hadn't been born into the Jewish tradition, I would likely have checked out how to join. I decided that no response was required from me because, by my own definitions, the appellation is true.

*

I was receiving my infusions at home every other week, without any side effect or other problem. These infusions were simply part of the twice-monthly routine, until late one afternoon. My home infusion company regretfully informed me by telephone, while I was in the checkout line at the supermarket, that my next dose, due in several days, had not been ordered from the pharmaceutical company. The caller informed me that they were very sorry.

Social courtesy would call for me to be gracious and accepting of their innocent mistake. Anyone can misstep unintentionally. Besides, no one really wants to be next in line behind some guy who is talking on his cell phone at the supermarket checkout. I ended the call quickly.

Wheeling my grocery cart into the parking lot, my thoughts turned to my history prior to the availability of enzyme replacement therapy. I ran through the chronology. "Well," I thought, "there was internal bleeding within an inch of my life, there was an acute hemorrhagic spleen, there were necroses, bone crises, and loss of bone mineralization, and there was a high grade malignancy followed by a severe infection, the combination of which cost me a leg."

And then I asked myself, "How important is it to me to be kind and accepting? Would I give my life for the sake of this social courtesy?" I concluded, "No, I do not want an epitaph that says, 'He was always kind to people even when their work performance was substandard.'" "No," I decided, "I need my medicine."

I called Patient Support at the drug company that was the manufacturer at the time of my Gaucher medicine. I explained the problem and my access specialist fully comprehended the situation. This issue wasn't as immediately urgent as post surgical pain or an icy driveway. But I had lost my reluctance to be selfish. I would require people who are responsible to me to stand for something. I was straightforward in communicating my expectation to the access specialist that my infusion would occur on schedule.

In whatever discussions occurred between the home infusion company and the drug manufacturer, the outcome was that my infusion occurred on schedule.

*

My in-laws were about to celebrate their sixtieth wedding anniversary. And they wanted this to occur in style. They wanted to create memories. A total of eighteen of us met in Miami to board one of the largest cruise ships afloat.

There were thousands of other passengers, but we made our own party. Among us were six cancer survivors, including my wife's cousin, Ann. She had survived a very nasty episode of breast cancer, and had elected for bilateral mastectomies. Early in the week we learned that there would be a Sexiest Legs Contest on Thursday, after departing from Saint Maarten. "Uncle Wayne, you have to enter that!" gushed Cousin Ann. I didn't respond. We had several days of fun, sun, and alcohol between then and Thursday. "Maybe Ann will forget by then," I thought.

Ann had a leadership position of great responsibility with a large manufacturing company. She had a mind for detail and the assertiveness and goal-direction required to manage a large workforce. Maybe there is a gene in my wife's family for lioness behaviors. Saying no to Ann was not an option.

It was immediately apparent on Thursday morning that Ann remembered. "Oh, crap," I thought.

The Sexiest Legs Contest would occur in the afternoon on Deck 11, the open-air Pool Deck. Deck 12 included the running track, which served as a surrounding observation point. The effect was a large amphitheater, full of scantily clad vacationers in a state of cruise-induced hypomania, and alcohol-induced disinhibition. This was an audience ready for a good time.

Ann and I ducked into a corner for preparation of my leg. She had brought a formal, black, lacy brassiere in which she had placed her pair of 34B prosthetic breasts.

"I should have bought some lace stockings in Saint Maarten," she lamented. "Oh, well," she concluded. "This will have to do."

She wrapped the brassiere's back strap a few times around my prosthetic leg. The cruise director walked by and her jaw fell open. "We're getting ready to enter the Sexiest Leg competition," Ann told her. We somehow conveyed to the cruise director that we were both cancer survivors. Ann demonstrated our plan for victory by giving the prosthetic breasts on my prosthetic leg a jiggle.

The cruise director held a microphone and sounded quite dignified as she introduced the contest procedure. Many people crowded the Pool Deck, and the rails of the running track on Deck 12 held many more. Somewhere in this crowd was Ann (she had a spare pair for the bathing suit), her husband, her children, my wife, my children, and the rest of my wife's extended family. I dared not look at the crowd out of fear of losing my nerve, or of falling down. Each contestant was required to somehow exhibit his legs to the three, very scantily clad female judges, who were volunteers from among the passengers. The other men each performed some sort of dance routine for the judges.

Introduced as "Uncle Wayne," I did a nonverbal improvised mime routine that suggestively compared the breasts on my prosthetic leg to the barely concealed breasts in the judges' bathing suits. It's a blur, but I think the crowd applauded. The judges were very good sports about the whole thing. One of them, whom I believe did not speak English, accepted my nonverbal gestural offer for her to touch the breasts on my leg.

After all contestants had performed, the judges conferred. There were several award categories, leading up to the top prize. The cruise director announced the awards to loud applause from the crowd.

"And the top prize, for Sexiest Legs, goes to... Uncle Wayne!"

The crowd erupted and cheered as I stepped forward, with my breasts still tastefully bobbling within the black, lace brassiere on my leg. Out of range of her microphone the cruise director said quietly to me, "I've never seen anything like this." Still dignified but now with a broad grin she brought the microphone back up to her mouth and added, "I think I should say too that Uncle Wayne is a cancer survivor." The cheers were louder yet. The cruise director placed a medal around my neck and a prize hat onto my head. I am told by my children that passengers were quietly pointing me out for the remainder of the cruise.

What happened that day at sea was a world away from staring at ceiling tiles in a hospital. I thought that this story was so off-the-chart inappropriate for a credentialed professional that I would never speak of it onshore. "What happens in the Bermuda Triangle stays in the Bermuda Triangle," I quipped.

Six months later, Ann learned that she had a metastatic recurrence of her breast cancer. There was still an experimental chemotherapy to try, but her options were limited. Ann spoke to me about her fear of being trapped in her body in great pain, and then of being unable to express herself.

Fourteen months after the cruise in which our combined cancer histories won the prize for Sexiest Legs, Ann was surrounded by her family. She was unable to move or speak. I held her right hand for a short time, while my older son held her other hand. I was reminded of the day when I held the hand of a patient in similar condition. I didn't know what Ann could hear or understand. But I said aloud that I knew that her fear was of being in pain at this point. Those present, all devoted to her comfort, agreed that she did not seem to be in distress.

With Ann's prior approval, in a place far from the Bermuda Triangle, I related our victory in the Sexiest Legs contest, in my eulogy at her funeral.

*

One summer Sue announced that we would be taking a vacation. Zion National Park and Bryce Canyon in Utah, and the North Rim of the Grand Canyon in Arizona, were on her to-do list. We would reach that part of the world by way of the airport in Las Vegas.

The Zion National Park experience is one of hiking within some spectacular natural scenery. Walking sticks are a part of the local custom among the hikers, so I brought out my cane. I was delighted to wear shorts on the trails, revealing the latest high technology, microprocessor controlled leg. We chose a trail through the woods that had a difficulty rating of easy to moderate. It had some low hills, but was wide and not too rocky.

A family appeared over a small rise, coming toward us from the opposite direction. The face on a young man in his early teens seemed to indicate that he was not enjoying this vacation option. I don't know what the conversation might have been before I saw them. But I heard the father say, "If he can do it, you can do it." I straightened up and walked a little more assertively as I passed them.

*

I regularly present a shortened version of my lifelong Gaucher Disease story at meetings for patients, as a contracted spokesman for a pharmaceutical company. I continue to have the impression, first developed years earlier, that the Gaucher Disease population's ability to cope is facilitated by social connections. These speaking opportunities allow me to meet many people with Gaucher Disease and their families, which is quite important to me.

During a connection in Atlanta during one such trip, I overheard airline employees in the terminal discussing the need for a certain airplane parked at the gate to receive maintenance, following "a hard landing." There had been no extraordinary weather in that area.

On this day, I was flying home to New England during a winter storm. I had a window seat on the left of the airplane, just in front of the engine. Late in the flight the pilot announced that we would experience "a few bumps" during our descent in darkness into our destination airport near Providence, Rhode Island. A science nerd knows things. And I knew that we would be lucky to avoid diversion to Boston or Hartford or maybe even further, because of the severe weather.

The plane bounced during the turbulent descent, as we had been warned. The landing light outside my window shined off the clouds revealing a steady stream of horizontal snow. The plane seemed to want to turn to the right, and then to the left. But it quickly seemed to nudge back. In an instant the clouds were gone and I saw that we were already close to the ground, passing the perimeter fence of the airport. There continued to be a steady stream of horizontal snow outside my window. The sound of the engines diminished and the feeling was of dangling over the airport. My nerd brain knew that, rather than dangling, we were actually moving forward at a speed faster than any car that I'll ever drive. Then part of the aircraft seemed to tentatively touch the ground. Then more of the aircraft was touching the ground. The aircraft seemed now to be showing more confidence as a vehicle that rolls rather than flies. The engines reversed thrust and outside my window was a swirl of white snow blowing in all directions. The cabin full of passengers broke into spontaneous cheering and applause during the extended roll almost to the end of the runway. We had witnessed the work of a professional as he fought chaotic winds and then a slippery, snowy runway.

Both pilots were still in their seats as the passengers exited. One passenger stuck his head into the flight deck to say something complimentary. But there was no other indication that anything extraordinary had happened. But I thought that what I had just witnessed in Rhode Island was indeed special. We did not just have a safe landing. We had a smooth landing.

I wrote to the airline's customer service department, commending what, to me, was a job performed with great skill. I've taught my sons that any job can be done well. But we expect aircraft pilots to always do their jobs well. Just as in graduate school, anything less than a 'B' is a failing grade. We also expect superlative performance in many other jobs. "Almost good enough" is not acceptable for a psychologist, a pediatrician, a policeman, a nurse, an anesthesiologist, or an orthopaedic surgeon. We just expect these jobs to be done well, and with integrity. Our civilized society depends upon this.

*

I worked many hours each week, because I enjoyed what I was doing. I performed Emergency Department assessments of very acute situations. I conducted group therapy on an inpatient psychiatric unit for people who met the stringent requirements of being a danger to themselves or others, or of being gravely disabled by a mental condition. And I provided individual therapy in an outpatient clinic.

I encountered very many people who were described as being suicidal. There are about a dozen risk factors for suicide, based upon one national organization that provides information and training for the professional community. These risk factors are counterbalanced by protective factors. The empirical problem is that all of these identified factors for risk of, or protection from suicide are statistically unreliable, just like horse races. These factors, so far, have not been translated into numbers that can be reproduced again and again. Although we know the overall risk factors, the assessment of suicide risk for any individual must rely heavily upon the skill of the diagnostician.

I thought of my old friend, the $y=mx+b$ formula, and how it expands to become the formulas for inferential statistics, the ways that science predicts the future. If we could have numbers of sufficient statistical reliability, then we could test people in the Emergency Department, do the arithmetic, and know who is at risk and who is not. But that is the fantasy of a science nerd. People are too unique and every situation is different.

I seemed to be good at suicide risk assessment. My colleagues and patients validated my judgment. I would occasionally run into people outside of the hospital who thanked me and told me that my assessments of their, or their loved ones' situations had been correct. That was nice to hear. It was a source of pride to me to know that situations were stabilizing and that lives that I had touched had been affected for the better.

Suicide risk assessment requires a great deal of knowledge. But a high quality assessment, one that is correct, rests upon the ability of a clinician to form a trusting relationship, evidence great perspicacity for subtle cues and to not become emotionally overwhelmed by the weight of the task. I often told my colleagues, "This is the most grownup job in mental health." The psychologist who was my first supervisor in this line of work explicitly instructed me to consider the needs of my patient above anything else. I was told not to worry about the cases that were waiting to be seen, or the need of the hospital to fill inpatient beds, or the need of the Emergency Department to move the cases along quickly. I was to do what I needed to do to reach a correct assessment. A correct assessment is one that neither hospitalizes people unnecessarily, nor releases people whose circumstances are in some way dangerous. I appreciated this directive very much. This fit with my personal values.

I identified with the struggles of people who were presenting with acute emergencies. I knew that, whether they said so or not, they expected me to be a professional who would put their needs above all else. They expected me to be smart enough to know how to perform their assessment. They expected me to care. They expected me to represent values that would help them.

I also knew the experience of being at the mercy of credentialed professionals. On some days in the Emergency Department I briefly glanced up at the ceiling tiles. The ceiling tiles are what a patient arriving in the Emergency Department sees first. And the ceiling tiles are there, looking back at patients waiting to be medically cleared, or waiting for the psychologist. I was aware too that, for patients lying in a bed and looking up to talk to me, the ceiling tiles framed my face.

One of the most important suicidal risk factors to consider in such an assessment is *hopelessness*. Depression would seem to be a more logical predictor. But, no, hopelessness is a greater risk factor. I would sometimes think about my terrible Thanksgiving Day, when I was at my most miserable. But I had hope on that day, that the doctor from the Pain Service would return, that he would not give up on me, and that I would be home, as he promised, for Hanukah. I met many people in the Emergency Department who had lost their hope.

I had seen the despondency and hopelessness of suicidal patients on many occasions. Even though I can intellectually understand that hopelessness is an important risk factor, I cannot fully appreciate the depth of despair that they must experience. I recall days of utter misery, but I have not been suicidal. I am no stranger to emotional distress. But with each victory I became stronger. Very often during an interview I would think, "How she must suffer."

*

In the emergency departments I would sometimes encounter the families of people who had lost someone important to them. I recalled how much I had relied upon my trusted professionals to make me well. Working in emergency services I was acutely aware that good outcomes are not guaranteed. There were people who did not survive their illnesses or injuries. And there were those who were successful with self-destruction. Even though I had a secret fantasy of being able to soothe everyone's pain and fix every problem, I was aware that life is not always gentle.

I saw the mother of a young man who died of a toxic ingestion. I don't know if his actions were suicidal or simply reckless. Trying to find meaning in his death his mother asked about harvesting his body parts for transplantation. My thoughts turned to my allograft. I was witnessing a scene similar to what must have occurred prior to the harvesting of the tissue that I was given during my cancer surgery. Perhaps this young man's death would provide parts for someone else's life, just as I received a donor bone. Sadly, this woman's beloved son died from ingestion of a substance that poisoned his body. His parts were unsuitable for transplantation.

*

In an outpatient clinic, I was involved in the identification and treatment of psychological trauma. A key component of the cognitive-behavioral treatment of posttraumatic stress is the development of the affected person's own trauma narrative. Trauma narratives can be very difficult to hear. The practitioners of this therapy place themselves at risk for all of the emotional and even physical problems suffered by their patients.

I found that I was very successful with the treatment of trauma. One of my adult patients gave me a tiny glass angel. She explained, "The angel is a symbol of peace, and you have given me peace of mind. I don't know how you did it."

A teenage survivor of trauma surprised me one day with a wood plaque into which she burned, "Dr. Wayne. The best psychologist ever." Recalling that I told my father that I would need to be among the best in this field, I cherish this gift.

I believe that part of my effectiveness with emergency services and trauma therapy is that I am not overwhelmed by extreme emotional intensity. But I am sufficiently accomplished in empirical methodology to know that a *single subject, posttest only* research design says practically nothing that can be generalized. This would be equivalent to saying, "We have a person and here is what happened to him." My successful adaptation to my own trauma narrative may not be good science. I wouldn't want to try to present my story at a dissertation defense. But it is the story of how I became good at this.

35.

I felt that I could hear descriptions of terrible things and not feel the need to withdraw from disturbing imagery or descriptions of recalled situations. I did not have a need to hear less. My trauma patients could relate their memories of awful things, and their psychologist could listen attentively and respond with a statement that conveyed understanding. I could help people to build their own trauma narratives, and to become desensitized to them. I appear to have become emotionally tolerant of extreme situations, immersing myself in them without becoming vicariously traumatized myself. Coming through what I have come through, I'm a better psychologist for the experience.

*

During the time that I was involved with trauma therapy in an outpatient mental health clinic, there was a terrible massacre of young children and their teachers in Newtown, Connecticut. My disaster mental health team was activated and the members were polled as to availability.

The bodybuilders at my gym could see the treadmill that I used for my workouts from where they were lifting weights. Some of them remarked that they felt inspired, and maybe a little bit challenged, by seeing me, with my high technology leg, performing an extended treadmill workout. To one of them I responded, "I don't have time to be disabled." I was on a treadmill the morning after the massacre when I received the telephone call to report to Newtown.

There are many parts to a disaster and many opportunities to experience intense emotions without any preparation. I spent time with a woman who had been traumatized by what she had seen and she cried intensely. By now I had a healthy respect for vicarious traumatization. Although this is a cliché, you really do feel another person's pain. I felt that I could have cried along with her. But I thought, "No, one of us has to be the psychologist here. And I'm the one wearing the badge with the big red PhD on it, so the psychologist will be me." I continued to give verbal reflection as she debriefed. After about forty minutes, I could see that she was becoming more comfortable. After an hour she announced that she was feeling better and would be leaving to go home. I had brought my tolerance for stress to bear on this situation. I hadn't reached my limit, but I could see it on the horizon. I was reminded not to try to be an emotional Superman.

*

A year later, the hospital where I was working participated in a large disaster drill. The scenario was that of a school shooting and involved many organizations that would be called upon to respond in such a situation. I was assigned to stay with parents in a special room away from the Emergency Department. According to the drill scenario, these were parents who believed that their children had been brought to the hospital, but who had no other information. I would be in contact by telephone with a colleague stationed in the Emergency Department.

I introduced myself to the parents, who were doing a very good job at being distraught and demanding. I asked everyone for their names and for the names of their children. I promised them that I would give them only factual and confirmed information. Knowing the names of the children whose parents were hounding me, I called my colleague inside the Emergency Department by telephone. She told me the names of the children who were known to be present in the hospital. I made a list on the sheet on my clipboard, but I tried to shield the names from the emotional parents.

These were the real-life parents of children who had volunteered to be a part of this drill, so there was a considerable sense of realism with their concern. My colleague called back and gave me the triage report for the children in the Emergency Department. "Amy has a sprained ankle from jumping out a window," she reported privately to me by telephone while I took notes. The parents studied my face for any reaction. "Jeff has a shoulder laceration. Jennifer has a gunshot wound to the chest and her condition is unknown." I started to feel panic as my colleague continued, "Debbie is in emotional shock but she has no physical injuries."

I was the only professional with these parents. I went down the list that I had, giving reassuring and helpful news to the parents of Amy, Jeff, and Debbie. Jennifer's mother was waiting for some news. "I need to call one of our nurses," I told her. I was starting to feel extremely overwhelmed. I called the nurse supervisor. "Natalie, would you come up to the family room? Thank you." I wanted someone else to be there with me, because I was about to tell Jennifer's mother that her daughter has a high caliber gunshot wound to the chest, which most certainly cannot be good. "She may already be dead," I thought, "depending upon the scripted scenario."

Before my professional backup could arrive, however, an announcement over the hospital speaker system informed us that the disaster drill was ending. An Emergency Department disaster drill ends when a non-drill serious case comes in. The Emergency Department staff would quickly turn their attention to responding to an actual emergency, perhaps saving someone's life for real.

The parents and I walked down the hall to a large conference room for the debriefing. Jennifer's mother told me that she suspected that something terrible had happened to her daughter, because she could see that I skipped over Jennifer's name on my list. Just then, the real Jennifer came in and hugged her Mom. She had a large quantity of stage blood on her chest. I told her that I was very glad to see her. "I mean, I'm *really* glad to see you!" I added for emphasis. Jennifer had no idea who I was or why I would say these things. As a test of my own emotional endurance, I felt that I had very nearly reached my limit. Finally, the nurse supervisor arrived, and I told her why I had needed her earlier. Fortunately, this was only a drill.

*

I had another one of the Gaucher Disease patient meetings scheduled for midweek. It would be a dinner meeting, about seventy-five miles from the outpatient clinic. I would be able to keep my regular work schedule that day, and still leave the hospital in enough time to arrive promptly for the meeting.

I was now the outpatient therapist for my previously suicidal emergency patient. She had missed several weeks of appointments and, when I did finally see her, I thought that she seemed depressed. She smiled faintly and denied any suicidal intent or plan. My recommendation was that we should get an immediate review of her medication. Her psychiatric appointment was scheduled for the next day. I quite plainly told her that if she did not attend her appointment

I would have the police check on her and, if necessary, have her brought involuntarily to the Emergency Department.

Late the next day the psychiatrist came into my office. The psychiatrist shared my concerns. But we agreed that the evidence was insufficient on which to base an involuntary admission.

Two days later I was within fifteen minutes of departure to my dinner meeting with Gaucher Disease patients. The psychiatrist entered my office. "We were both right about her mood," she said. The patient had survived another suicide attempt. The psychiatrist told me that our patient had just been transferred to the inpatient psychiatric unit, and asked if I would see her.

I swiped my badge at the entrance to the psychiatric unit and heard the door unlock electronically. Opening doors is still satisfying after all these years. I found the patient sitting on her bed.

She had again ingested an overdose, with the intention to die. Instead, the chemicals caused unexpected changes in her behavior and mental status. "It was terrifying," she said.

I told her that I couldn't stay long because of my scheduled talk in about an hour and a half. While I was sitting with her my cellular telephone rang. It was one of the writers involved with me on a revision of my Gaucher Disease presentation.

"Is this a good time to talk?" asked the voice from far away.
"Not really," I said. "I'm on the inpatient psych unit. Working."
My patient laughed. I completed the call quickly.

"You'd better get going," my patient admonished me, "or you'll be late for your talk." She thanked me again for visiting her and promised me that she would be safe. I had heard that same promise earlier in the week, but I was glad to hear it again anyway.

She would eventually be my patient again in the clinic. We discussed her frustration with a chronic mood disorder that seemed to be a lifelong challenge. In some ways, I thought, a mental disorder is worse than what I have been through. It seemed to be a lot harder for her than for me, to create distance between her disorder and herself as a person. I had endured a sick spleen, a damaged hip, and a very sick leg, all of which I was willing to remove from myself, while I continued to see the rest of me as healthy.

My patient and I developed a plan together for cognitive behavioral treatment of her distress. I tried to convey to her my own genuine feelings of hopefulness regarding her future. I didn't promise her an easy solution. But I did tell her that an improvement in her emotional situation is possible. I know the importance of hearing hopefulness from a provider.

36.

I'm declaring victory. The future continues to unfold, often in unforeseeable ways. Man plans, and God laughs. But right now, I'm declaring victory. I won. My life after cancer, and with regular enzyme replacement therapy, has been remarkably full and busy. I'm having the time of my life.

A *shofar*, the hollowed-out horn of a male goat, is blown in the synagogue on *Rosh Hashanah*. Trumpet solos are a distant undergraduate memory. My last trumpet gig was with the Alfred University Jazz Ensemble. But I found that I can pick up one of these horns and fill the room with the blast. Some of my most treasured compliments are those that I have received from Holocaust survivors and from survivors of the Soviet Union's attempt to eradicate Jewish culture. The families that remained in Eastern Europe into the late twentieth century are very emotionally demonstrative. Some of them have broken traditional synagogue decorum to applaud.

*

My sons, Aaron and David, the little kids who pushed the button on my morphine pump, have grown into fine men. Their Dad is not just an abstraction. I have survived to be an influence in their adult lives and to share in their successes. They have seen me endure horrible experiences and have seen me adapt to the realities. They have not been vicariously traumatized, because they have seen me cope, fight, and win.

They too have adapted to the realities. On one occasion, when they were still very young, we were all flying from Connecticut to Florida, by way of a tight connection in Pittsburgh. David knew just the right words to use to prod me along: "Dad, walk the way you do when you're mad at us!"

And they have learned to assert themselves. On another flight to Florida the stewardesses were selling airplane cookies. These are like animal cookies, but in the shape of airplanes. Aaron was next to me and I asked him if he wanted some cookies. He declined. The stewardess with the rolling cart passed and was somewhere behind us. Aaron then decided that he would like to have the cookies. "It's too late," I told him, and he didn't get the cookies.

He asked if he could play with my smartphone and I handed it over. Months later I found a note on the smartphone: "A good Dad would buy me cookies."

*

Sometimes I need to laugh at the utter absurdity of the situations in which I find myself. On one trip to Florida, David and I were in a kayak in an inland portion of Tampa Bay. Then, for some reason that I don't recall, we were in the water, out of the kayak. I observed my partially buoyant aqua-leg near the boat. "David, would you grab that?" I requested. Don't you just hate it when your parts start to float away?

*

On one *Yom Kippur* eve Sue and I were getting ready to go to synagogue. I used the hex wrench given to me by my prosthetist to change the dorsiflexion of my foot so I could wear formal shoes. I must have loosened too many of the screws simultaneously. The foot with the formal shoe fell out

174

of the pylon and hit the floor with a thud. My wife's deadpan response: "What happened? Your foot fell off?" It had been her idea to see *Airplane!* during the days prior to my dissertation defense, but now we were living a scene better suited for *Beetlejuice.*

She expanded on that theme one day as she cleaned the attic while I was at work. Sue's wedding dress had been sitting there for decades, neatly packed in a storage box. She spread it out on the bed to discover that it bore a striking resemblance to the wedding dress in the spirit conjuring in *Beetlejuice.* With no prior warning I encountered it when I returned home. I expected to see it rise, containing Mrs. Maitland. I hurried to the den. "There's a scene from *Beetlejuice* in the bedroom," I gushed.

*

When my son Aaron was completing his degree requirements in Italian Language and Culture, he needed to spend a semester in the ancient city of Siena, Italy. His lioness mother suspected that Aaron was becoming homesick. With the words, "One of us has to visit him and your schedule is more flexible than mine," I was ordered to Tuscany. I flew to Galileo Galilei International Airport, in Pisa, which is an ironically hilarious destination for a science nerd. Aaron had grown by years in the few months that he had been away. He performed all of our logistical functions in Italian; ordering our lunch, getting a cab for us to the Leaning Tower, and buying our transportation tickets to Siena. I was thrilled to see him blossom into a respected and competent adult. And, just like the exploding chandelier in the prologue of *Phantom*, I felt blessed to be able to see it.

*

Both of my sons have learned determination in achievement of their goals. David announced one day that he was training to run a marathon. I know that a marathon is a grueling race, twenty-six miles and three hundred and eighty-five yards. Another bit of trivia I learned in college is that the first runner from Marathon to Athens did so in full armor, after the battle, proclaimed, "We are victorious!" and died. I reminded David, "We have a family tradition of — oh, what's the word — overdoing it!" I pointed out to him that his grandfather didn't just join the Masons, he became a Master. And he didn't just join a synagogue, he became its president. He would have been Potentate of his Shrine temple if he had lived a few more years. And I reminded David that his own father didn't just get a college education, he finished a PhD.

But David wanted to complete a marathon. He knew the significance of his name as the victor against a large enemy. He knew his father's liberal use of this metaphor in defeating the *angiosarcoma*. The date of the marathon was close to the twentieth anniversary of my amputation, my final battle to defeat the cancer. Recalling my fear that those young boys would never know me as adults, I told David, "I'll be at the finish line." "So will I," said the twenty-four year old.

I brought David and his college friend and running partner to the starting point in Austin, Texas before sunrise. The runners each carried tiny timing chips, transponders similar to those used for toll-collection on highways. As David crossed each timing mat, the app on my smartphone would show me his time, and the estimated time of his finish. There was nothing else for me to do but wait, as he churned through the streets of Austin.

About a half hour before David's projected time of completion I found a spot near the festive archway of the finish line. David had passed the timing mat at twenty miles. There would be no further updates until he arrived at the finish line.

The time of his projected finish passed and there was no sign of David. I received a text message from him informing me that he was within three miles of the finish, but his knee hurt a lot. I texted back "Don't hurt yourself. There will be other marathons." I wanted him to know that commemorating my victory anniversary was not worth an orthopaedic injury and that I would not be disappointed in him if he needed to quit for the sake of his wellbeing. Then I heard nothing more from him. I know David to be tenacious and very, very goal directed. Finally, his friend's sister yelled, "There they are!" And there was David, hobbling uncomfortably on a wrapped knee. We high-five'ed just seconds before he crossed the final timing mat marking the finish. Another commitment had been met.

*

Aaron was accepted for a six-month internship in Israel. I had been studying Hebrew for several years and I was ready for an opportunity to be on the streets in Israel to use what I had learned. I offered David the opportunity to run in the Jerusalem Marathon. It was fun to speak Hebrew in Israel with Aaron. I was able to go to the Western Wall with both of them. And I was again at the finish when a modern-day David conquered Jerusalem, completing another marathon.

*

I followed my science nerd instincts into amateur radio. I decided that the entry level, Technician license was all that I would need. I would be licensed to do all sorts of interesting things with that license, including the opportunity to play with satellites again, for the first time since college. I attended classes for several weeks. Before the completion of the course I felt that I was ready to take the examination. On a Sunday morning I drove to a testing session. I gave my completed answer booklet to one of the examiners and sat down to await the result. He walked over to me with another booklet and said simply "Here. Try this one."

"Oh, crap," I thought. "I must have failed and he's giving me another crack at it."

I looked at the questions on the second test. These questions seemed to be more difficult. And I didn't recognize some of the material. I looked at the cover page. "Oh, I get it." The second test was for the General class license. Now I realized that I had passed the Technician test. I had an opportunity to parlay that success into a General class license, which offered greater frequency privileges, including those for long-range communication. I missed a passing score by only two questions. "Do you want to try again?" "Sure," I answered.

I must have taken all of the available forms of the General class license, always missing a passing score by only one or two questions. "But," I reasoned, "that was without reading the book." So I bought the General Class License Manual and studied one chapter each week.

I found an examination session and passed. The examiner asked me if I would like to try the Amateur Extra test. This was a hard test. I didn't even come close to passing. "But," I reasoned again, "that was without reading the book."

"Oh come on," I thought. "Do I need to get a PhD in this too? Can't I just have fun with it?" Unlimited access to all of the amateur radio frequencies, global license reciprocity, bragging rights… I was powerless; the draw was too great. I bought the Amateur Extra License Manual and started reading. I took the practice tests at the end of each of the early chapters and I seemed to be doing acceptably well. Then the material became more difficult. I finished chapters without having the faintest idea of what I had just read. I thought, "This is nuts. I'm trying to teach myself to be an electronics engineer. I have reached my intellectual ceiling."

My wife asked me how it was going. "It's hard," I said. She couldn't understand why I would continue with something that was no longer fun. But I did not want to admit defeat. I found online practice tests, and I began to pass one out of three. I found an examination session and I failed the test. I asked to take another form of the examination. This time I passed.

To communicate through amateur satellites, or to talk to an astronaut on the International Space Station, all I really needed was the Technician class license. I have a recording of an astronaut acknowledging my call sign and telling me, "We have you loud and clear aboard the space station." This recording is the best possible nine-seconds of audio for a science nerd.

*

I believe that most survivors of any major illness or traumatic experience would say that their lives were changed by the events. To the extent that this story exists as a trauma narrative, it is my experience with Gaucher Disease, a single misplaced nucleotide on the long arm of chromosome one. As an ancient rabbi famously said many years ago, "The rest is commentary." I survived some truly terrible things. I learned that everyday life can be cruel. And I learned a few things about what it takes to survive. I think I developed some skill with it. The most meaningful change is the appreciation that comes with victory. Since surviving all of the trials that ended in 1993, the air smells a little fresher, and many seemingly inconsequential daily occurrences have greater meaning. And the joys and successes seem to be more intense.

My experiences as a patient, a connoisseur of ceiling tiles, taught me what consumers of services need. They need integrity. They need to know that the professional truly cares about them. And this cannot be faked. The way to make people think that you care about them is to really, genuinely care about them. The way to make people think that you have integrity is to act with integrity. As consumers, we should expect nothing less from our providers. And our providers should already be acting this way. They should be standing for something.

I characterize my infusions, tests, and other medical experiences simply as my support for everything else I want to do. On one occasion I was preparing for a presentation and I shared my graphics with David. He asked me why I list paying taxes and insurance premiums as one of my life's valued activities. The answer I gave him is that paying taxes and insurance premiums is part of a normal life. This would not be the activity of someone staring at the ceiling tiles. I have a photo from a family vacation in which both David and I are helmeted, in a dune buggy. The people in that photo are enjoying being a part of life.

My life is not as a patient. As my prosthetist taught me years earlier, the prosthetic leg is a tool to allow me to participate in everything else. He told me that a clean and shiny prosthesis belongs to someone who is not using it to be a part of life. The enzyme replacement infusions are another such tool. Life is with the people and activities that give meaning. I was so thankful that I could see the chandelier explode again in *Phantom*. I was thankful to see Aaron's ability to speak and live in different cultures. I was thankful to see David cross the finish lines. Mostly I am thankful to see them grow into fine men, honest, compassionate, and dedicated to doing a great

180

job in whatever they want to do. I have seen some of the best and worst examples of professional behavior. And I am thankful that my own life experiences, some painful, some academically challenging, can combine to allow me to contribute meaningfully to the lives of others.

Every two weeks I receive a delivery of my enzyme replacement medicine. My nurse contacts me during the evening to confirm the delivery. Then she arrives at my home in the morning. We exchange pleasantries and chat about the things we have in common. She starts my intravenous line, and mixes the medicine. When all of the drug is mixed and injected into the bag with the saline, she starts the flow. We talk, she measures my temperature and blood pressure, and we talk some more. When the intravenous infusion is complete, she removes the line from my arm, packs up her supplies, and we confirm the next appointment. And that is my current Gaucher Disease experience. There is no sensation or discomfort or any outward indication of a physiological effect of this medicine.

I will occasionally remark to a provider that I have a terrible Gaucher Disease story, but not a single serious Gaucher Disease manifestation since 1993, when I began to receive these infusions. In much of the world people like me still suffer and die. But in the United States this seems like distant history, an abstraction for how Gaucher Disease once affected people, including me.

I survived many terrible experiences during the time before enzyme replacement therapy. During the years of my Gaucher Disease narrative I've met many people with similar stories. And I have known a few of the people who did not survive. Unlike the military officer with whom I worked in the middle school, or even the medical students who have heard my lectures or felt my spleen, people with Gaucher Disease did not choose to participate in their challenges. We did not volunteer, we cannot resign, we had no training and, when we see the ceiling tiles en route to the operating room, we are completely alone. We may have much support and encouragement from those around us, but there is only one person living inside each of our bodies. In each individual case, it's our fight. With Gaucher Disease, or with any chronic or acute illness, we are alone to fight the Wicked Witch, the Klingon cruiser, or the uncircumcised Philistine.

I improvised my survival at every point. Only in retrospect did I appreciate the importance of an internal narrative of coping and strength, and the importance of properly visualizing the goal of survival and success. Along the way I saw the importance of social connections and mutual support among people fighting the same enemy. We now also have the benefit of success stories, and I will be very pleased if my story is one that conveys strength to someone who needs it.

Bringing my experience and lessons to bear on the problems of others gives meaning to what I have endured. When I achieve each new diagnostic or therapeutic success in my own work, I see what would not have happened if I had not survived. The physical and psychological components of my narrative have forced me to clarify what is important to me, to stand for something that I find meaningful, and to selfishly demand what I need and is properly mine. I have asserted myself personally when necessary, and have been unabashedly confrontative at times. For myself and for those around me, pain is not to be ignored, and professionals will not be devaluing or self-serving. Professionals are expected to act with integrity and to be worthy of our trust. I have been radicalized by my experiences.

This is my path to being a psychologist who can properly evaluate emergency, disaster, or traumatic conditions, and to be the person in the right place, with the right credentials, knowledge, and emotional fortitude to willingly immerse myself in extraordinarily intense situations. This is my path to being capable and motivated to help people, to professionally stand for something. My professional path includes my Gaucher Disease narrative, which has demanded a great deal of emotional fortitude.

We had some homegrown heroes in Massachusetts. One of my personal favorites is a woman who managed the house, the farm, and the family while her husband was in Europe seeking financial backing for the American Revolution. Less than a century and a half after that scary Puritan started a settlement ninety miles west, this lioness chose to inoculate her children for smallpox, at a time when the procedure itself was highly unpleasant and could be deadly. She held her eldest daughter's hand during the young woman's surgery without anesthesia for an advanced breast cancer.

She and her husband agreed that their young son should accompany his father when he returned to France. The child saw this as an unwelcome disruption to his life in Massachusetts. But his mother insisted that young John Quincy Adams would accompany his father, John Adams, to France. The boy sailed to Europe with his father. He learned many things, and he adopted his parents' values. At that time no one could have foreseen that he would someday be the US Ambassador to Russia, and that he would chat in French during morning walks with the Czar. No one predicted that he would be a President well regarded by history. No one could have predicted that he would someday be recalled from retirement to appear before the Supreme Court in defense of the prisoners of the *Amistad*.

Abigail Adams had a worldly wisdom regarding the conditions that cultivate psychological growth. And her advice to John Quincy is relevant to so many of us today:

"It is not in the still calm of life or the repose of a pacific station that great characters are formed. The habits of a vigorous mind are formed in contending with difficulties. Great necessities call out great virtues."

Acknowledgements and Thoughts

I wonder if Philippe Charles Ernest Gaucher stressed about defending his dissertation, in the days when physicians needed to demonstrate their empirical skills in the traditional manner, even without award of a PhD degree. His *post mortem* description of the young woman who seemed to have a nonlethal leukemia started the scientific inquiry into this bizarre disorder.

The story of the development of a treatment for Gaucher Disease is a scientific adventure story spanning decades. The ability to target an enzyme to the membrane of a microscopic structure inside cells has saved many lives, including mine. I was present at a meeting of the National Gaucher Foundation when many people who could not walk just a few years earlier, pulled themselves to their feet to applaud one of the key researchers for the development of a Gaucher Disease treatment.

Dr. Henry Mankin, the Gaucher expert who sentenced me to years of walking on crutches during high school became my greatest hero. He is like another father to me, although his jokes are better than those of the guy who married my Mom. I met many of the orthopaedic surgery residents and fellows who studied under his direction. I saw him as a professor who demanded that his residents and fellows in orthopaedic surgery demonstrate at least his own level of skill, and was thrilled when he saw them give even more. One student who missed the significance of my splenectomy scar received an immediate and intense remedial lesson.

My prosthetist continued to ensure that my mobility was nothing worse than inconvenient, until his retirement. I last saw him at a farewell dinner prior to another trip overseas to make legs for children in far away places.

During the last hours of his life my Dad still spoke of how proud he was of me. He gave me his personal values.

I visited my Mom at her skilled nursing facility almost every week for about sixteen years. She wanted to be a part of the research at the National Institutes of Health into the relationship of the n370s mutation to Parkinson's Disease. However, her health made travel from Boston to Bethesda impossible. She pragmatically gave me permission to make proper *post mortem* use of her brain and other parts, if doing so would help others. Regarding her brain she told me, "I won't be using it at that point." The tissues of greatest research interest were harvested by a neuropathologist in Boston and were then sent to a research laboratory at the National Institutes of Health. The vigilant mother who watched over me during my worst times wanted to contribute in any way possible to our knowledge of Gaucher Disease. She continues to participate in research on our behalf.

My friend, predoctoral research collaborator, and Best Man, Sheldon Klein, became an extremely well respected psychologist. He sold the horse. We believe that she was eventually auctioned at an event for retiring trotters and pacers. Our understanding is that she spent the rest of her life pulling the buggy of an Amish family.

My wife Sue has been my loyal companion and partner starting with my dissertation defense and then through the numerous later medical decisions and surgeries, and beyond. My cancer story did not occur in isolation. There was a household and two young children to care for, compounded by the emotional and physical workload of a sick husband. She did it all, and she was my greatest advocate and guide through the worst of it. I don't know where she found the strength.

I enjoy visiting the campus of Alfred University, where I have a memory associated with many of the buildings. I have also had many opportunities to revisit the campus of the University of Connecticut. The dormitory looks the same, where I and other doctoral students led solitary lives together. There is now a huge indoor sports stadium where I used to park. And the complex is within sight of the library where my dissertation is on a low shelf in the basement.

I received invaluable editing and other advice for the production of this story from Kay Norlander, PhD, a former research assistant who was later a professor. She retired from academia, but she is still my sister-in-law.

I also received editing assistance from David Rosenfield, who prodded me to include additional details and triumphs that needed to be shared.

I met my old friend, Abby Turner Schwartzlow, at a recent Gaucher Disease patient meeting. Together we told her husband the story that culminated with our dance. Abby told me that her last bone crisis occurred while she was in college, more than ten years ago. Then Abby whispered to me, "I'm pregnant." Abby later helped me to confirm certain information for this narrative, including my father's emotional response to her first infusion. Abby was multitasking, because our communication occurred while she nursed her beautiful daughter. She's another one of life's participants.

I know that my story is just one of thousands of possible narratives from people with Gaucher Disease and any number of other chronic conditions. Everyone's story is different, although they are similar in some important ways. I have also met very many people with disorders of feeling, thinking, learning, and behavior, and I appreciate the intense distress that they sometimes endure.

My wish for all who are living with chronic disorders is that they will only encounter providers whose intelligence and devotion are worthy of them, and that they will stay strong.

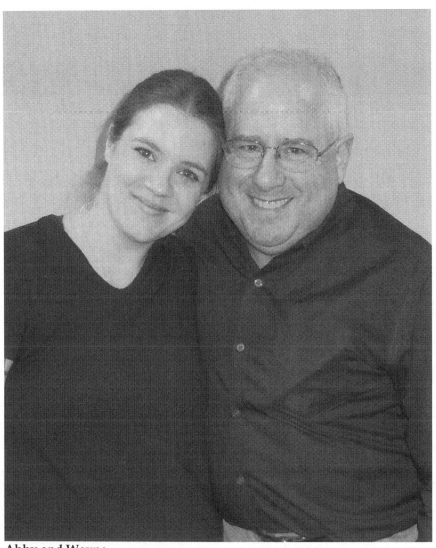

Abby and Wayne

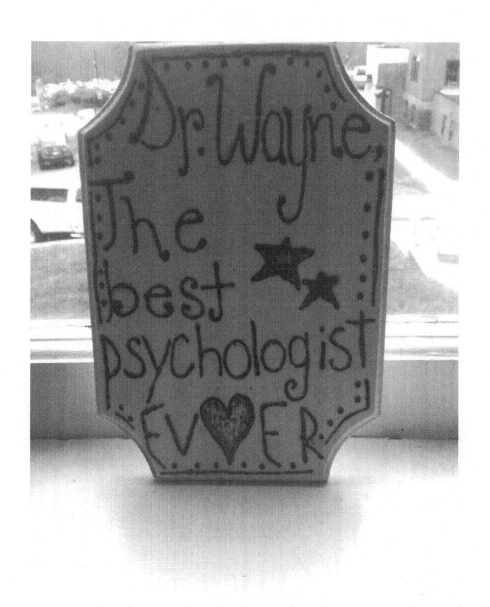

A surprise gift from a young survivor of trauma.